KETO DIET

Over 50

THE ULTIMATE AND COMPLETE GUIDE FOR HEALTHY WEIGHT LOSS, SLOWING AGING AND PREVENTING DIABETES WITH KETOGENIC LIFESTYLE.

+ 10-DAY MEAL PLAN WITH 30 LOW-CARB RECIPES

Amanda K. Loss

-Table of Contents-

INTRODUCTION

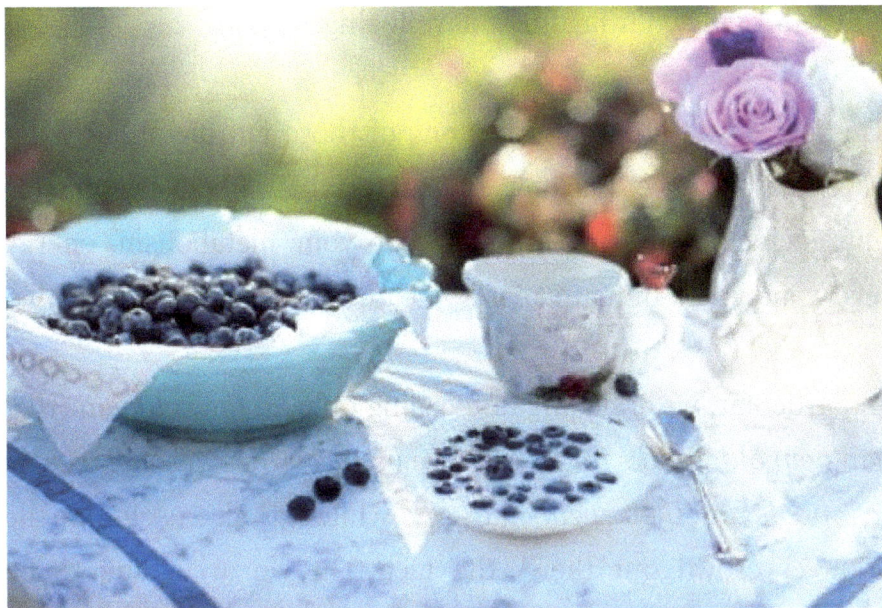

Thank you so much for choosing this book *Keto Diet Over 50*. We will show you how to make your Ketogenic diet journey amazing and hassle-free.

If you are reading this, it is because you are keen on learning more about how you can improve your overall health and wellbeing while dropping some pounds along the way. So, this book has been written with you in mind. It doesn't matter where you are coming from. What truly matters is that you are concerned about improving yourself.

In this book, you will find tips and strategies regarding the use of the ketogenic diet as a means of losing weight, feeling better, and improving your health and wellbeing.

This book isn't about another one of those fad diets that don't have any science backing them. It is all about a sensible approach in which you can improve your metabolism, energy levels and your ability to keep some unwanted extra pounds off.

In particular, we are going to focusing on *how the ketogenic diet can help older folks find a balance between their overall weight loss goals and their wellbeing*. And while it is also useful for the younger crowd out there, the fact that we are going to be focusing on the ketogenic diet for older folks makes this book highly specialized.

So, what are you waiting for?

Come on in and let's get started today on your personal journey to improving your health and wellbeing!

CHAPTER 1: WHAT IS THE KETOGENIC DIET?

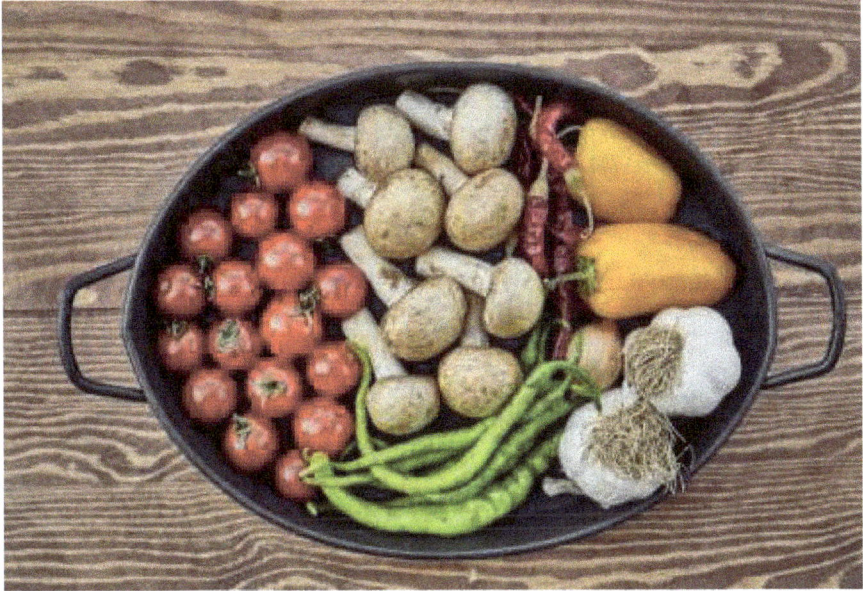

Hundreds of years ago, what we ate did not matter that much because we were healthy as we only ate natural foods available. However, over the decades, the food industry transformed, and food companies started introducing food additives and chemicals to food to increase its taste and shelf life.

This transformation resulted in an increase of diseases previously unheard of in ancient times. In this book, you will learn what this diet is, how it works, its benefits, and how you can adapt it to have a lean body, free from excess fat and live a healthy life. Obesity becomes one of the scariest words in the modern world. Being overweight has become an annoying problem. Many people are trying to lose their weight by following many kinds of dieting methods. Since an ideal bodyweight and a healthy body condition are significant concerns nowadays, the diet has become a trend in the new community.

Many people have tried many dieting methods with all of their hard treatments. Even, some people are willing to pay handsomely to reach the ideal bodyweight. You might have heard that a Ketogenic diet is a dieting method that has been effective for the last several years. It is also known as a Low Carb Diet.

Principally, the Ketogenic diet involves a high intake of fat, moderate consumption of protein, and tremendously low eating of carbohydrates. In other words, it can be said that the Ketogenic diet is a dieting method that encourages the liver to produce more ketone bodies. Lucky you, this book provides many recipes that will help you to prepare excellent and healthy food! In this book, you will learn valuable and critical information on how you can use the Ketogenic diet to lose weight and better your health.

The Ketogenic diet is a diet that focuses on reducing your carbohydrate intake and makes you eat more healthy fats. It is also a diet that has been proven not only to help lose pounds but also to control significant medical conditions like epilepsy. In the following chapters, we will explain exactly what the

Ketogenic entails, how it is different from other diet plans, the benefits, and some helpful guidelines on what to eat and what to avoid when living a Ketogenic lifestyle. This book will teach you everything you need to know about the Ketogenic diet, how it works, what foods to eat, what foods to avoid, and how you can get started. This book also contains a starting 10-day keto meal plan that can help guide you through your very first phase. Starting a keto diet can be tough if you don't have a good idea for what to eat. That's where this 10-day keto meal plan comes in. We've done all the calculations, cooking, and planning for you. Now you can relax and enjoy all the benefits of a Ketogenic diet stress-free. Thank you again for believing in us and getting started. I hope that you will enjoy it and that it'll help you along your journey to more excellent health.

I am so excited that you have chosen to take a new path using the Ketogenic diet plan. The plan is recognized by several names, including the low-carb diet, Ketogenic low-carbohydrate diet & high fat (LCHF) diet plan, and the Keto diet.

Your liver produces ketones, which are used as energy to provide sufficient levels of protein. The process of ketosis is natural and occurs daily – no matter the total of carbs consumed.

Before you begin the journey to ketosis; here is a bit of insight on how the diet plan was discovered:

During history, as early as the 20th century, fasting was theorized by Bernard McFadden/Bernarr Macfadden as a means for restoring your health. One of his students introduced a treatment for epilepsy using the same plan. In 1912, it was reported by the New York Medical Journal that the fast is a successful method to treat epileptic patients, followed by a starch- and sugar-free diet.

In 1921, Rollin Woodyatt noted the liver produced the ketone bodies (three water-soluble compounds, β-hydroxybutyrate, acetone, and acetoacetate) as a result of a diet low in carbohydrates and rich in fat.

Also, in 1921, Dr. Russell Wilder, who worked for the Mayo Clinic, became well-known when he formulated the keto plan, which was then used as part of the epilepsy therapy treatment plan. He had a considerable interest in the project because he also had epilepsy. The program became known for its other effects, which helped in weight loss, and many other ailments.

The ketosis dieting technique was set aside in the 1940s because "improved" methods were discovered for the treatment of epilepsy. However, during that time - approximately 30% of the cases using the alternate plan failed. Therefore, the original Ketogenic plan was reintroduced to the patients. As of 2016, Wilder is still functioning successfully without the seizure episodes.

As a direct result of Dr. Wilder's discovery, innovation began at the Mayo Clinic. Another physician standardized the diet plan using the following calculation:

- 10-15 carbs daily
- 1 gram of protein per kilogram of bodyweight
- The remainder of the count will remain with fat

As time passed, the plan had a few changes to make it functional as it is today.

The family of Charlie Abraham founded the Charlie Foundation in 1994 after his recovery from seizures he had daily, and other health issues. Charlie—as a youngster—was placed on the diet, and he continued to use it for five years. As of 2016, he is still functioning successfully without the seizure episodes and is furthering his education as a college student.

The Ketogenic diet has been utilized for 92 years as a weight loss diet and a means of controlling certain medical conditions. We are going to take a look at the basics of the Ketogenic diet to show how it can work for you today. The Ketogenic diet is a low carb diet that contains a moderate amount of protein, low carbohydrates, and high-fats. The Ketogenic plan focuses on reducing the percentage of carbs eaten to force the body to break down fats instead. The keto diet was made specifically for you to reach ketosis. Ketosis is a metabolic state where your body produces ketones. Ketones are provided by your liver and are used as fuel towards your body and brain instead of glucose. To make ketones, your diet must be low in carbs and only an adequate amount of protein. The Ketogenic diet is often compared to other foods like the Atkins diet and the Paleo diet.

While both the Atkins and Paleo diet's focus on cutting carbs down, there is a significant difference in how each plan uses this reduction in carbohydrates. The Ketogenic diet relies on deficient levels of carbohydrates to put the body into a state of ketosis throughout the entire menu. This enables your body to continue to rely on fat-burning rather than sugar (glucose) burning for energy. The Atkins diet relies upon a lack of carbohydrates in the initial phase of dieting but then reintroduces carbs gradually at lower rates. The paleo diet, however, can or cannot be Ketogenic because it does allow for the consumption of starches. Additionally, the paleo diet does not necessarily have to include higher levels of fats like the Atkin's, and Keto foods do.

One other way that the Ketogenic diet stands out from other diets is because it has a medical application for individuals with epilepsy. Research has shown that higher levels of ketones in the blood have been proven to reduce seizure activity. So the Ketogenic diet has applications for those with epilepsy or other seizure disorders. Usually, you get your energy from glucose, but on a Ketogenic diet, your body switches its fuel source to burning fat. When this occurs, your insulin levels will be low, and you will be burning fat always. Many people can safely follow a Ketogenic diet. Still, in some situations, you should take a more logical approach; for example, if you have diabetes, high blood pressure, or breastfeeding, you should research for alternatives. Since the Ketogenic diet changes the way that your body metabolizes nutrients. It is essential to check in regularly with your primary physician or dietitian.

Regular checks will help you to ensure that you are maintaining sufficient levels of nutrients and not pushing your body over the limits. It should be noted here that at ANY time you are considering a new diet plan, you MUST check in with your primary physician or dietitian! A quick check will make sure that a dietary plan like the Ketogenic diet is safe for you based on your current body mass as well as with any other existing health conditions.

Types of Ketogenic Diets

There are four main types of the Ketogenic diet, including:

Standard Ketogenic Diet (SKD): This is a very low-carb moderate-protein and high-fat type of diet. The standard food contains 75% of fats, 20% of protein, and only 5% of carbohydrates or less.

Cyclical Ketogenic Diet (CKD): This diet involves a period of high carb refeeds, for example, five days where you eat Ketogenic, followed by two days where you eat high carbs.

Targeted Ketogenic Diet (TKD): This diet is meant for athletes or those who exercise daily. It is where you eat mostly Ketogenic and high carbs during workouts.

High-Protein Ketogenic Diet: This is much like the standard Ketogenic diet; the only difference is that it includes more protein. The high-protein diet contains 60% fat, 35% protein, and only 5% of carbohydrates or less. Throughout this book, we will only be focusing on the standard Ketogenic diet. But if you hold much interest in the other Ketogenic diet versions, feels free to study them extensively.

Some Side Effects to Lookout For

Now the truth is, if you are not used to the Ketogenic diet, you might notice some side effects from it. Many people get demotivated after they follow this plan, simply because they don't feel like this plan will do them any good. However, let me assure you that these things will go away very quickly, so you don't have to worry about it. The first thing you will notice would be the keto flu. Many people who follow the Ketogenic diet tend to get sick in the first week. Which is fine, as it could be a part of the food. There is no explanation as to why people get sick within the first week, but it is something that happens. Make sure you take some time for recovery before you jump back on a diet. The second thing you might notice would be that throwing up would occur from time to time. This will only happen in the first few weeks, against freak out as many people experience this. The reason why an individual might throw up is simply that they are not accustomed to the high-fat diet. Keep that in mind, and if it makes you feel any better, have some carbs after you have thrown up. One of the significant side effects you might notice is nausea or even feeling like fainting if you feel like that, please make sure you have a look at your food consumption. Having an understanding of how much you are eating, especially on a Ketogenic diet, is very critical. Make sure that you are eating enough, as some people under eat when following the Ketogenic diet, overall, be cautious of this. Hunger is something you will notice when following the Ketogenic diet. Please note that the Ketogenic diet will only make you feel the excessive desire in the beginning once you get accustomed to the food, it will go away. The last side effect you will notice would be bad breath. Please note that the bad breath will go away eventually. However, in the beginning, you will have a metallic smelling breath. Feel free to have some low-carb gum and water to combat this issue. Lemon water with no added sugar works the best if you can handle the sourness.

Chapter 2: Benefits of the Ketogenic Diet

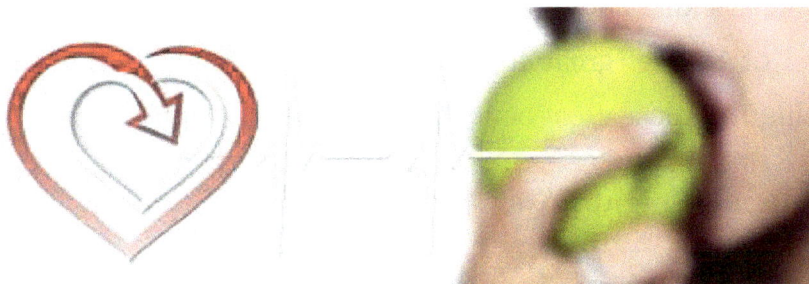

The most apparent benefit of the Ketogenic diet is, of course, weight loss. While you will find that any food can help you lose weight if you cut enough calories, the Ketogenic diet is explicitly optimized for fat loss. If you've been struggling to shed a spare tire or you've wanted to whittle your waist, the Ketogenic diet may be just what you've been looking for. But how exactly does the Ketogenic diet work for weight loss? The concept is relatively simple. When you reduce your carbohydrate intake so that your body no longer has stored glucose to burn for fuel, it has to find something else to consume. In addition to burning the fat you eat, your body will also start to hack away at your stored fat. Numerous research studies have shown that the Ketogenic diet is much more effective in burning fat than low-fat and high-carb diets. The body needs fats as raw materials to produce ketones for fuel! In addition to increasing fat burn, the Ketogenic diet will also reduce insulin production, so you stop storing fat. That means that even if you do overeat once in a while, you're not going to undo all of the progress you've made with the diet. You will also find that the Ketogenic diet reduces your appetite, so you feel less hungry between meals, and that will help keep you from snacking and overeating. All of the above is fine and dandy and of course, great to hear, but what exactly is the science behind all these great benefits and more? Let's find out!

Natural Weight Loss

This is pretty much one of the main drivers for many; many folks are taking up the Ketogenic diet, and at least I know I was also one of them, hopping on the bandwagon when I knew I needed weight loss in order to improve my health situation. The Ketogenic diet is really great for weight loss, as you will soon find out when you embark on the meal plans and really get into ketosis. The true magic of this is that you engage your body to help you out in losing the weight, instead of relying on calorie counting and restrictions to generate fat burn. When we first start out on the diet, we will begin to lose water weight in the initial stages. The reason for this is primarily due to our stored carbohydrates being present in mainly liquid glycogen form. As we reduce the reliance on carbohydrates, the body draws down upon these easily available stores of energy first as it grapples with the transition into ketosis. This water weight loss can account for anything from 5 to 20 pounds, depending on your initial starting weight when you begin the keto diet. This is a great morale booster to be sure, and most folks credit the keto diet with the lost weight. If we were to be very exacting in our specifications though, this water weight loss is actually due to us restricting our carbs rather than the actual process of fat-burning ketosis.

As we get beyond the first few days and transit into the first few weeks of being on the keto diet, that is when further drops on the weighing scale will definitely be recorded. The key here is the carbohydrate restriction that we have been constantly harping on. As a source of quick fuel, carbs can be second to none. The glucose obtained from the carbs channel quickly into all areas of the body and provides them with the necessary energy boost when needed. The downside for this is that our bodies aren't really built for storing carbs. We really cannot store beyond a day or two of energy unlike our fat stores. When we cut down on carbs, the body goes into ketosis as we all know by now. This nature's alternate plan for energy would see fats being processed through the liver and then converted into energy-giving ketones. That is also part of the reason why some folks actually term the Ketogenic diet as a starvation diet.

In a sense, they are not wrong, because this alternate way for the body to produce energy actually can sustain a human for up to a month without ingestion of food. The fat stores become the fuel for energy. However, I would definitely have to state most strongly that we are not starving ourselves whilst on the keto diet. Just because ketosis is nature's way of not letting us starve when we are deprived of food does not mean there should be any negative connotations attached to it. More importantly, whilst on the keto diet, we have to remember that we are not really counting calories and it is a definite must to eat when we feel hungry.

When our body successfully transits into burning fat for fuel, this would mean the stored fat as well as the fat that we consume daily would become fair game for ketone production. The trick here is the need to let the body get accustomed to burning fat instead of glucose, which is the main reason why the keto diet is a high-fat low carb diet. As long we do not break ourselves out of ketosis, the weight loss that we experience would definitely be from the fats, aside from the initial water weight loss mentioned earlier. No exercise, no calorie restriction, no weight pills and exotic berries which you need for losing weight. The Ketogenic diet simply enlists the body's natural functions in order to kick start this powerful process of natural fat loss, however this only works if you are obese; workouts will be shown later. One thing to note however, this does not mean that you get to eat and binge all the way.

No matter what methods you use to lose weight, if you were to overeat and consume food even when you feel satiated, I would dare say it would be a tall order to instigate any weight loss if that were the case. Happily, there is something about the Ketogenic diet that also helps to prevent overeating. Read on!

Hunger Management

First off, when we wean ourselves from the carb-based diet and move on to a fat-based one, we are already doing ourselves a favor when it comes to hunger management. Carbs generally call to their own, like the sirens of yore that sailors in ancient times feared so much. Tell me if you have experienced this. You finish a bag of chips or perhaps three chocolate doughnuts, and within an hour or two, your stomach growls a little and there is that little, warmish feeling at the pit of your belly signaling that it is about time to find food again. The primary cause of this would be due to the blood sugar fluctuations happening whenever there is an over the top intake of glucose. We would be talking more about this in the later segment, but it would suffice now to say that when we transit to a primarily fat-based diet, this issue with the carbs meddling with the feelings of hunger will go away. As we move into ketosis and the body activates the fat-burning process for energy, we would generally feel less instances of hunger and more feelings of satiety. This occurs even if we were to be eating just two meals in a day, which I must say, is quite common amongst keto practitioners. As we take in more fat and moderate amounts of protein, these two essential macronutrients have the ability to let you feel satiated and get that feeling of fullness for longer periods of time than if you were on a carb-based diet.

Couple this with the fact that the majority of processed and unhealthy foods have plenty of carbs in them, it shouldn't come as too much of a surprise that you would start feeling less hunger as you cut out these empty calories and replace them with nutrient-dense whole foods consisting of fat and protein. Beyond this, being in ketosis actually causes a double whammy effect on the hormones that control hunger pangs. Ghrelin, the hormone that makes us feel hungry, sees its production being muted when our body is in ketosis. This is good news because ghrelin usually increases whenever we engage in any traditional dieting and start losing weight. This would mean that you would be stuck in between a rock and a hard place. The more you try to lose weight via conventional dieting, the more hunger you would feel due to increased ghrelin production! Besides this, the hormone that controls the feeling of satiety, cholecystokinin, experiences a complete reversal of what just happened to ghrelin whilst the body is deep in ketosis. Typically, as you lose weight, cholecystokinin production decreases in a bid to induce you to eat more. However, ketosis prevents the levels from dropping even when the body is experiencing weight loss.

This works out very well for anyone who is on the keto diet because we get spared the hunger pangs that usually accompany traditional dieting. Some have actually asked if this would mean that the body may potentially waste itself into nothingness since feelings of hunger are suppressed and we may not know if we are truly hungry. To answer this, we would first have to come to an understanding that the body, as an organism, is a wonderful, intricately balanced piece of self-learning machine. The ability of the body to sort itself out is virtually second to none. When we are in ketosis, we will still experience hunger as our energy stores run down through expenditure via daily activities. These feelings of hunger are what I would consider as true hunger, as they are not created from a carb induced state of affairs. When you feel such hunger on the Ketogenic diet, it is usually a very strong signal to get your next meal! At least that is what I always do. That is why many keto practitioners always talk about eating only when you truly feel hungry and not be subjected to the usual social norms of eating during breakfast, lunch and dinner times. It really can feel quite liberating to be in touch with your body's needs. So, the idea that we would gradually waste away to nothingness really does not hold much water because we still would get signals of hunger to prompt us to eat. What really happens is that we get these hunger pangs less frequently than if we were to be still on a carb-based diet. The adjustments in the produced levels of hunger controlling hormones do play their part, as do the satiating feeling of fats and proteins. There is also another reason for the less frequent hunger pangs. We simply are getting more energy from the fat-burning!

More Energy and Mental Clarity

I am quite sure that I am not alone in having the experience of feeling weariness or even fatigue just after a meal heavy in carbs. Just imagine having had a hearty meal, perhaps even topping it off with a nice, sugary dessert, and literally within the hour you find yourself nodding off, scarcely able to keep your eyes open despite your best efforts. I know my many instances of bruised thighs can attest to how hard I pinch myself trying to keep awake.

The thing here with this fatigue is that it can be easily avoided if you were to cut down on carbs! When the body breaks down carbs for fuel, the glucose generated needs insulin to act as a mediator in order to be transported into the various organs and cells to be used as energy. That is primarily the reason why our pancreas jacks up our insulin production whenever we have a carb-heavy meal. The body knows that it needs to safely usher the blood sugar present in our bloodstream to be used as energy or to be converted and stored as fats. In cases where our bodies are fairly young and not metabolically damaged, the resulting insulin sensitivity is still high, and the pancreas is able to create just about the right amount of insulin to match the level of blood sugar present. However, as we age and damage our bodies metabolically through inattention and diet, our insulin sensitivity decreases, and this leads the pancreas to produce ever-increasing amounts of insulin in order to ferry the same amount of blood sugar. The poor pancreas realizes that the body's cells aren't responding like they are previously to insulin and hence increases its production as a way to normalize the situation. This then results in a swift reduction of glucose in the bloodstream which triggers the tiredness.

If we give in to the fatigue and quickly go to bed, you might realize that we often wake up with a roaring hunger, which is also coupled with a strange feeling of bloated-ness in the stomach. When there is low blood sugar in our bodies, the body triggers hunger signals in order to get additional fuel. The bloated feeling in the stomach though, is a result of food not being fully digested. If we think about it, a hearty lunch should let us feel satisfied all the way until dinner time in normal circumstances. Why is it that we get feelings of hunger and fatigue just a few hours after our last meal? The key lies in the fuel that powers our bodies. Glucose triggers the insulin response, which in turn has the potential to create the so-called sugar crash that causes the tiredness and accompanying hunger. Energy-based from sugar or glucose can be compared to a candle's light, flickering and winking, subject to the whims of the wind. When your body is energized by ketones however, this power source is akin to an electric bulb, shining bright steadily and consistently.

When our bodies burn fat, insulin is hardly called into action. This limits the sugar crash possibility. Also, as fat is easier to store and more readily available than glucose in our body, the ketones produced from fat can readily draw upon our body's fat stores. We get a stable source of fuel as a result, which then explains why we feel more energetic on the keto diet as compared to a regular one. Ketones also provide more bang for the proverbial buck as compared to glucose, as they burn cleaner, metabolically. When you place a plentiful source of fuel and couple it with the fuel's better energy-giving capabilities, is it any wonder that you probably would feel like being able to handle all the work and house chores, and still have energy for that special project which you have always been wanting to embark on? The buck doesn't stop here though. You may think having increased energy from the keto diet is really a great benefit. How about getting improved mental clarity to boot? Say goodbye to those days of fuzzy headedness and times when you just cannot seem to concentrate and be ready to embrace life with razor-sharp mental alertness.

What really happens behind the scenes to account for the boosted mental acuity, is the effect of ketones on the brain. Our brain hangs on the balance of two major neurotransmitters, glutamate as well as gamma-aminobutyric acid or otherwise known as GABA. Glutamate serves as a stimulant and is usually associated with intelligent processes, like talking or thinking abstractly. Geniuses are found to have higher levels of glutamate. Too high a level, without the balancing effect of GABA, would result in over-stimulation of the brain. This is when seizures, strokes and generic neurodegeneration occurs. As it turns out, glutamate needs the presence of the calming GABA in order to head off the potentially debilitating effects of over-stimulation.

What ketones does for the brain is to provide a more efficient way for which glutamate is processed into GABA, which then leads to a neural environment that has fewer neurons firing all at the same time. This translates to a real-world effect of having better mental clarity and doing away with brain fog. The brain also appreciates ketones as a better fuel. While it has to be said that it does require some amount of glucose to maintain a healthy function, this amount of glucose can be easily provided for via the limited carbs we take in as well as the process of gluconeogenesis, which is the creation of glucose via proteins. The difference between glucose and ketones as fuel can be markedly attributed to their oxidative footprint. Glucose, in excess, induces far more oxidative stress than ketones. Factor in the fact that the brain is literally a glucose hog while we are off the keto diet, and you have a case where it is a matter of when, not if oxidative damage would harm the brain. With the presence of ketones however, this oxidative damage is somewhat curbed and sometimes even reversed, leading to postulations about the neuroprotective qualities of ketosis.

Boosted Brain Health with Keto

You might have encountered instances where you have read about how the Ketogenic diet was used since the 1920s to help treat folks with epilepsy. It has been shown to reduce the incidence of seizures without the need for medication. In fact, treatment of epilepsy through dieting has long been espoused by the ancient Greeks. Hippocrates, the famous physician, was one of the forerunners of this therapy where medicine played a decidedly secondary role. Various research and anecdotal evidence have pointed to the efficacy of the Ketogenic diet in reducing or even totally suppressing seizures, particular in cases of childhood epilepsy. Recent medical research has postulated that the reason for these apparent benefits is mainly due to the increased energy production in the hippocampus, brought on by the introduction of ketones as fuel for the brain.

The increased energy levels found in the brain were thought to contribute significantly to ensuring more stability in neuron activity. The research also showed that the Ketogenic diet actually improved the brain's oxidative stress resistance, which bodes really well for other neurodegenerative diseases like

Alzheimer's and Parkinson's. Alzheimer's disease has been dubbed the diabetes of the brain, because the brain cells become insulin resistant and hence aren't able to receive their required amount of glucose. This deprivation of blood sugar to a glucose hog like the brain essentially means that fuel for neural processes is lowered; sometimes too much, and it leads to neural system damage. This then paves the way for Alzheimer's to take root. With the brain fueled by ketones however, insulin resistance of the cells can effectively be remedied, because there is very little need for insulin without reliance on glucose as fuel. Ketones also seem to provide an added layer of protection against oxidative damage.

For diseases like Parkinson's and certain types of dementia, oxidative damage to the brain cells, coupled with a lowered neural energy production, are thought to be the main culprits in letting these diseases take hold. When your body is in ketosis however, these two damaging factors are put on hold due to the presence of ketones. Another thing to consider is the impact of the additional fat that the Ketogenic diet introduces on the brain. The brain is effectively made up of about sixty percent fat.

There are tons of more benefits, but this should give you an idea of what the Ketogenic diet could do for you.

Chapter 3: Side Effects and Do's and Dont's

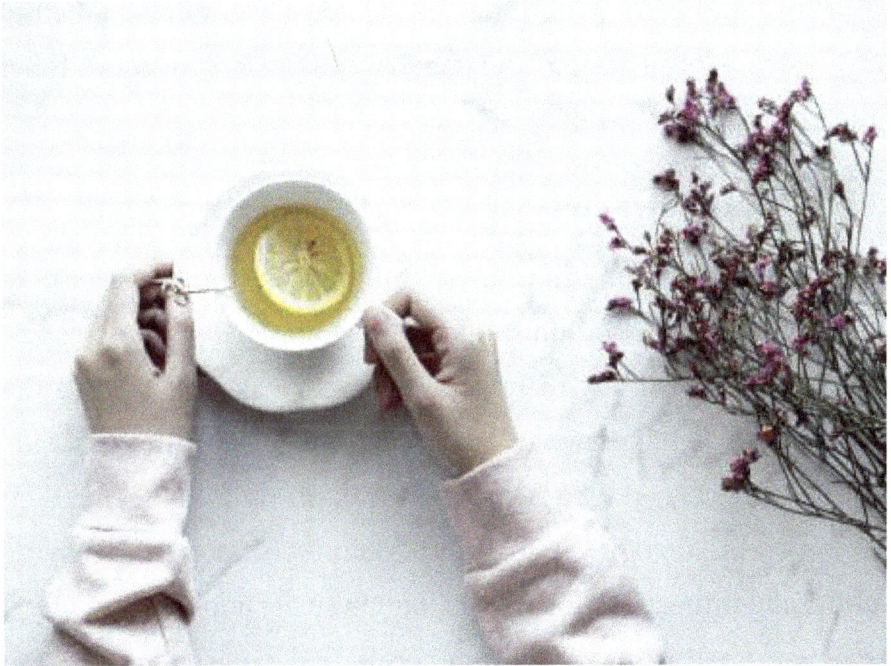

Now, you can easily understand why you are feeling the way you are after starting the diet and how you can control these side effects. What you really have to understand is that you are completely changing the way a normal body works and produces energy when you convert to a Ketogenic diet. It is quite normal for your body to resist the new change that you bring to it. But if you quit the gym on your first day because your body starts paining, chances are you are not going to go back to it any time soon. Some of the side effects that you may feel when you start a Ketogenic diet include the following: Urination - After the first day or two, you will notice that you are being forced to go to the bathroom to urinate more often. This happens because your body is trying to burn the last bits of glucose that is stored in your liver and body. When the body tried to break down glucose, it releases a lot of water. This is what makes to run to the toilet more often.

Fatigue and Dizziness

When you start urinating more, you will also end up dumping minerals like salt, sodium and magnesium as well. Having low minerals in your body will make you feel weak and dizzy in the first week or so. Fatigue and dizziness are some of the first side effects experienced by a person starting off on a Ketogenic diet. However, the flow of these minerals can be countered by having additional minerals in your food. Salt is easily added on any food that you are taking and for minerals like potassium, you can have dairy food, vegetables and avocados.

 Low Blood Sugar: Since your body might be used to getting high carbohydrate food before you transitioned to a Ketogenic diet, you might have bouts of Low Blood sugar. This is only natural, as your body is used to putting out insulin to counter the sugar that gets released by the intake of carbohydrates. This sudden change in your diet is what your body reacts to when you have low blood sugar. However, this will start to wear off when you are 2-3 weeks into the diet.

Constipation

Constipation is another common side effect of being on the Ketogenic diet. This is generally caused because of dehydration, loss of minerals, eating too much dairy or nuts or in some cases because of magnesium imbalances.

Sugar Cravings

As your body starts getting used to burning fats to fuel your body instead of sugar like it was used to earlier, you will start craving food with high carbohydrates. This is typical to last anywhere between 2-21 days. If you can fight the temptation, you will see that this craving will eventually start decreasing and then completely go away after a few weeks. It is essential that you do not consume any high carb food during this duration because it will stop the whole process of ketosis. Diarrhea is another typical side effect of being on a low carb diet and it should go away naturally in a few days. This especially occurs if you start eating low fat along with low carbohydrates which results in a greater intake of protein. Ensure that you substitute the carbohydrates that you are cutting down on by increasing the intake of fats, preferably saturated fats like butter or coconut oil. To help you out of this issue, you can try to take a tbsp. of sugar-free Metamucil or plain psyllium husk powder before you eat a meal so that the fiber absorbs the excess water in the colon.

This should help resolve any issue that you might have with diarrhea.

Shakiness or General Weakness

Both shakiness and general weakness are a side effect of low blood sugar, which sets in as you begin the Ketogenic diet. You can counter this by adding more protein to your diet and include foods that contain potassium. Alternatively, you can also take a 99mg supplement of potassium citrate. Sleep Deprivation People who are on a Ketogenic diet often complain about sleep deprivation. This may be because of low levels of insulin and serotonin in your system. To help with this, you can try to eat a snack, which contains both protein and some carbohydrate right before bed. The insulin will increase with the intake of carbohydrate and this will enable more tryptophan from the protein to flow to your brain. This will in turn facilitate the production of serotonin, which helps in having a calming effect on your brain. Another reason for losing sleep can be low histamine tolerance. Low carb diets are rich in histamine, which makes some people anxious and deprived of sleep.

Kidney Stones

A lot of people who argue the use of the Ketogenic diet, sight this as a compelling example of why one must not follow this diet. This is generally based on the formation of kidney stones among children who are suffering from epilepsy. But that comparison is actually not very accurate. For starters, the diets given to epileptic children contain close to 90% fat and the shakes that are given to such children are made of processed powders like Ketocal. When you are on a Ketogenic diet based on real food, your body receives some amount of protein. Furthermore, there are reports to suggest that a dose of citrate supplement can deter this from happening among epileptic children as well.

Low Thyroid Levels: This side effect is also argued as one of the negatives of a Ketogenic diet. However, that is only a natural response to a Ketogenic diet where your hunger is reduced. This same issue also arises when you are on a calorie-restricted diet made up of food rich in carbohydrates.

Racing Heart

A lot of people complain about having heart palpitations when they are in a Ketogenic diet for a few weeks or months. This is generally attributed to people with low blood pressure, although there are several other factors that might be responsible too. This include the lack of nutrients in the system, which can be provided by the use of a multivitamin and magnesium supplement. It could also be that the person is resistant to insulin and the low carbohydrate diet results in hypoglycemia. Having homemade mineral water along with your breakfast and evening meal can help if this is the issue. Some people can have a racy heart because of the over-use of coconut oil and MCT (medium-chain triglyceride) oil. When you add these to your diet, it is advisable to first start with limited quantities and increase the intake over time. It is also advisable to not only rely on coconut oil and MCT oil as your fat source but also include other fatty foods like butter, ghee, olive oil as well as animal fats.

Even though a Ketogenic diet allows for some intake of protein, depending on the individual, it may not be enough for them and they might have to increase the protein intake. Increasing the intake of protein by 5-10 grams each day can help in such a case. Hair Loss: There have been reports of people saying that they have experienced an increase in the amount of hair loss since they started a Ketogenic diet. However, this is natural in case of any change in diet and is not only restricted to a Ketogenic diet. This process of losing hair due to a change in metabolism or hormone levels is called "telogen effluvium." The lowering of insulin at the start of a Ketogenic diet is a normal but temporary side effect that could be a cause of hair loss among some people.

Low Carb Flu or Keto-Flu

As soon as you reduce the intake of carbohydrates to your body, suddenly you start feeling all the symptoms of the flu – headaches, dizziness, crankiness and exhaustion. We have gone through these separately in the points above, but a combination of all these might feel to some people as if they have caught the flu, without really feeling sick. As soon as you start reducing the intake of carbs, you start feeling an urge to stuff yourself more carbohydrates. This is because of something known as metabolic flexibility.

This is a problem that only some people might face. Metabolic flexibility is a process through which your body can change its source of fuel from carbs to fats without any problem. If you, for example, have a potato with butter, your body will first breakdown the potato into glucose and use it power your body; and when that is over, it will start breaking down the fat in the butter. But some people have impaired metabolic flexibility, which makes them cranky as soon as all the carbs in the body have been converted to glucose for energy. Their body instead of reverting to burn fats for energy, crave more carbs. If you eat a snack at this moment, your body will again use the carbs in the snack to power your body and all of the butter that you had eaten will get accumulated in the body as fats. It is almost certain that these flu-like symptoms will not last and will go away in a few weeks, but some of the things that you can do to fix this include: Take in the appropriate amount of carbs.

Do not shut them off permanently. Keep taking the amount that you calculated as per your lean body mass or ideal bodyweight. A lot of the symptoms are related to the deficiency of minerals and salts in your body as you start a Ketogenic diet. You can get help on these my taking in more electrolytes. It is also important that you ensure that you are taking in enough fats as per your body mass index. It is impossible to run a human body only on proteins, and if you keep insisting on your body using only protein as a primary source of energy, your body might just stop metabolizing and you will end up feeling starved as you have to take in enough calories. It is important to substitute the lowering of carbs by increasing the intake of fats in its place. A lot of studies have shown that exercise can help restore your metabolic flexibility but that can be a little hard to do when you are running out of steam 2 minutes into the exercise. If you can fight through the initial few days of these flu-like symptoms, you can start exercising after they are gone. Drinking plenty of water is extremely important when you are on a Ketogenic diet because when your body undergoes ketosis, it loses a lot of water and minerals initially. This causes dehydration, which gives rise to headaches. It is important to note that not everyone who starts a Ketogenic diet goes through this "low-carb flu." In most cases, there could be separate incidents of headaches etc. that can be countered using the methods mentioned in the points above. Most people who are metabolically flexible will never even experience such problems. And even if you do, wait and be patient. This is only temporary and will eventually go away. As you can see, we have listed a number of side effects that people generally complain about when they start a Ketogenic diet. But most of these are only natural and can be countered by simple measures that have been documented in the points above. The ideal thing to do is to weather as much of these side effects as you can, because they are all temporary and will generally go away after a few weeks.

As we have discussed many times over in the course of this book, it is natural to find limitations in your body as soon as you start a Ketogenic diet. But as your body starts adapting to the use of fats as an energy source, you will see that your strength and endurance will soon start coming back to normal. The question to ask yourself is this: does carbohydrates enable us to build muscle? And the answer to that question is: No, it doesn't. It is still possible to refill the glycogen levels in your body when you are on the Ketogenic diet. The key to that is the amount of protein that you intake. If that part of the diet is taken care of, you can put on body mass even when you are on a low carb diet. What you can do if you are specifically looking to put on more body mass is that you increase the intake of protein by 1 to 1.2g per lean body mass. It is true that putting on body mass during the Ketogenic diet is slow, but it is only because the total fat content of your body is not increasing as it is getting burnt to provide energy.

People often misquote that the Ketogenic diet makes you lose performance. But reports suggest otherwise. A recently concluded test on trained cyclists who were on a low card diet for 4 weeks showed that they retained the same muscle mass as they did before they started the diet and there was no dip in aerobic endurance either. Over the course of the diet, their bodies adapted to the process of using fat as an energy source, while limiting both glucose and glycogen stores. Another study conducted on eight gymnasts also seemed to yield the same result. In the case of both groups, they were fed green vegetables, proteins and very high-quality fats. Therefore, this proves that even when you are doing long bouts of cardio, the Ketogenic diet will come across as a hindrance for you. An exception to this could be an exercise where you are required to do an exercise that needs explosive action. To boost your performance during such an exercise, you can help yourself to 25-50 grams of carbohydrates, 30 minutes prior to starting the exercise. You can follow the following steps to know how to exercise when your body is in a state of Ketosis. Resistance training is a great way of building muscle as well shed fat and it does not require you to put in long hours at the gym to do so. You can try lifting in short but intense sessions to fasten the fat burning in your body. It is advisable to train in shorter sets. The number of repetitions in sets should ideally be limited to 10 and repeated numerous times instead of continuing for a long time. The short intervals in between the sets can be utilized by the body to build up any glycogen that it might have lost during the set.

Cardiovascular exercises are ideal exercises to perform when the body is in a state of Ketosis. Although a lot of people will advise against it, eating a small measure of carbohydrates after a workout session enables the sugar contained in the carbohydrate to travel directly to the muscles. If you find that you are not getting the desired results that you expected from your low-carb diet, it just might be that you are committing some of the common mistakes that people tend to make when on a Ketogenic diet.

Intake of Too Many Carbs

While this is one of the most common mistakes, this is generally the cause when you do not do proper research about how much carbohydrates are supposed to be enough according to your body mass index or ideal bodyweight. A lot of people think that anything under 100 grams per pound is enough for you to be able to produce enough ketone bodies to power your body. However, as we looked in an example before, with an ideal bodyweight of 150 pounds, ideally the most about of carbs that you should have is 30 grams only. Only when the carbohydrates are low enough will the body be able to switch from using carbs to power your body to using fats to power your body.

Intake of Too Much Protein

Protein is one of the most important micronutrients that the body needs to function optimally. Generally, having protein-rich food increases fat-burning. However, when someone is on a low carb diet, gorging on meat can end up increasing the intake of protein in your body. When the body consumes more protein than is required, the protein gets converted into glucose through a process called gluconeogenesis. This glucose gets broken down into sugar that gets used as fuel in your body instead of the fats. This breaks the ketosis state that the body is in. Too Little Intake of Fat A human body gets the greatest number of calories from the intake of foods rich in carbohydrates. If this source of calories is taken away, then the body will be starved of food to create energy out of. Some people, however, think that since having less carbohydrates is supposed to be good, so must be the case with having low fats as well. However, that is one of the biggest myths.

Without carbohydrates the body needs some source of nutrients to use as fuel and that is when it switches to burn fats into ketone bodies, which does not happen, if the number of fats being consumed is also low. If the carbohydrate and fat, both are taken in lesser amounts, the body will soon run out of energy and starve. As long as you are keeping away from trans-fats and from vegetable oils, there is no reason for you to be fearful of fats.

Low Sodium Levels

As soon as the body starts going into a state of ketosis, the insulin levels in the body start going down. One of many uses of insulin is that it is able to signal the fat cells to store fat, and similarly, the kidney to retain sodium.

When you are in a Ketogenic diet, your body will start losing water and other minerals including sodium and this is one of the reasons many complain about dizziness, weakness etc. in the first few weeks of starting a Ketogenic diet. This is because sodium is one of the most important electrolytes that are required by the body for it to function optimally. The best way to work around this is by taking additional sodium in your food. One of the best sources of food is salt and increasing the intake of salt is one of the best ways of countering this shortage of sodium in the body.

Impatience: Another common mistake, which is very often repeated, is being impatient with the process of ketosis. By default, the body is designed to accept only carbohydrates as a source to fuel the body. So, if carbs are available to the body, it will always take preference over any other source as a form of energy. When you stop the intake of carbohydrates suddenly, the body needs to get used to burning fats for energy instead of carbs. And it might take a while for the body to primarily burn fat for powering the body. During this period, as the body gets used to the new source of energy, it is very normal for the people undergoing this diet to feel dizzy or sick. Most people get alarmed as soon as they start feeling under the weather a little bit, and resort to discontinuing the schedule and diet as planned earlier. It usually takes anywhere between 2-10 days for the body to completely adapt to this new mechanism of burning fats. This requires you to be patient with yourself and trust the diet that you have planned for yourself.

Chapter 4: Ketogenic Diet for Younger People vs. Older People

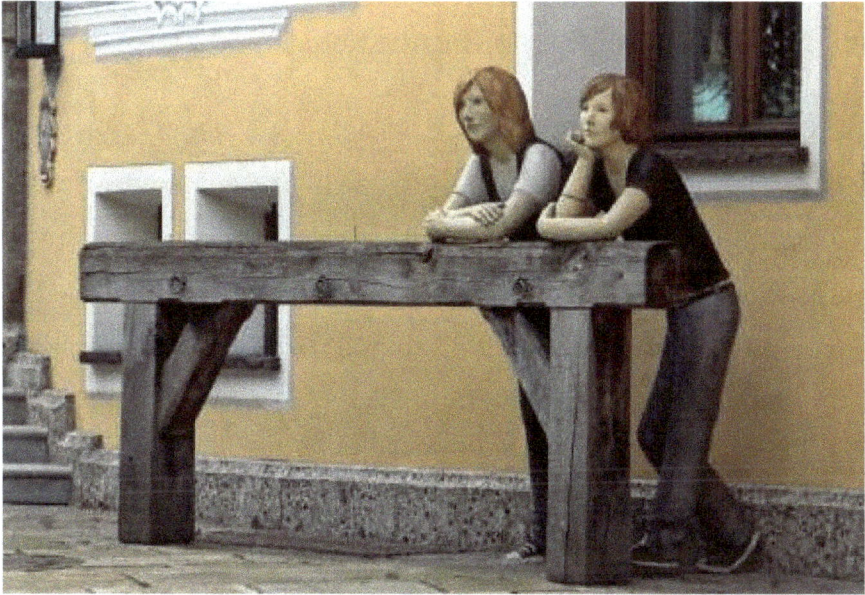

People think that it is because it is complicated to follow in the beginning. We have explained to you what the Ketogenic diet is and what it can do for you. However, it is your job to understand how it affects your body. Time and time again, many people who are above the age of 50, have seen amazing results with the Ketogenic diet. The reason is because they've seen such amazing results of the benefits; we have talked about the advantages which come along with Ketogenic diet, and they are very similar to the intermittent fasting benefits, which is why it is essential to understand that the Ketogenic diet can be a great asset to older people. Now don't get me wrong, the Ketogenic diet is for every age group and every sex. However, it is essential to understand the difference behind older people following the Ketogenic diet and the younger people following the Ketogenic diet.

The bottom line is that the Keto Diet is all about getting to ketosis. Therefore, for seniors, this will present some unique challenges, because they are not in the same physical realm as someone who is in their 20s. As a result of this, seniors need to think about the way that they do things, so that they can get the best possible results from the Keto Diet.

The good news is there are plenty of ways that seniors can use the Keto Diet and the process of ketosis to get some fantastic results. Actually, for seniors, there are many great benefits to ketosis, especially when it comes to keeping their minds sharp and their bodies active, so using the Keto Diet is something that will really invigorate many people who are seniors that are also healthy enough to take on the challenge of the diet. For seniors that miss the planning and the goal setting of working life, this is a great substitute because it engages so much more than the body.

There are many different things that come with old age, but just because you are getting older does not mean you should automatically be getting sicker. The bottom line is there is a connection between your aging and your health, and having a good diet is a great way to make sure that you are getting the most out of your senior years. In fact, when it comes to getting older, your diet is the easiest way for you to keep your vibrant and exciting lifestyle. As you age, there are several different ways that you can make sure that you are in optimal health. With that in mind, it is important to see the different things that ketosis brings to the life of seniors and how it is quite helpful. One of the things about aging that is impossible to reverse is the decline in our ability to do a variety of things.

We just simply are not able to run as fast as we once did, jump as high, and these physical limitations are something that is really impossible to reverse. That being said, if you are taking in a diet that has high carbs, all that you are doing is exacerbating the different problems that can be occurring within your body; therefore, the Keto Diet is a great way to make sure that you are not putting yourself that much more behind the 8-ball. Getting older is not a reason to mourn, though; you can become a healthier and happier person and maintain a greater level of physical health as you age than when you were younger. This is why the Keto Diet is so popular with seniors. It provides many different ways for seniors to support their health and get a greater quality of life than they would if they followed the same diet from when they were decades younger.

This is perhaps the best part of being a senior on the Keto Diet – better health as you move forward. There are several different benefits that come with being healthy and staying in ketosis as you go ahead and embark upon this diet. Understanding these effects and how they can help you is a big reason why seniors will benefit greatly from the Keto Diet and being in ketosis.

Resistance to Insulin: Unfortunately, there are many senior citizens who are considered overweight or obese, and they are dealing with conditions that relate to insulin such as diabetes. The problem here is that diabetes can impair you in a ton of ways such as getting kidney disease, diabetic neuropathy, necrosis, and even things like vision loss. When you are in ketosis, this removes blood sugar from your system along with insulin, which is a great way to cut down on the effects of diabetes.

Bone Health

One thing that many seniors struggle with is the health of their bones. As seniors age, one of the biggest issues they deal with is osteoporosis, meaning that their bones become brittle. This is especially common among women and that means that a fall could end up being something that would be much more severe than it would have been just a few years earlier. The reality is that drinking more milk is not the healthiest thing to do, because lactose operates the way carbohydrates work in the bodies. There is a correlation too – countries that have the largest rates of osteoporosis are also countries that have the highest rate of dairy consumption. That being said, ketosis works in a different way. There are tons of micronutrients that go right to your bones instead of blasting them with calcium. These micronutrients fortify the bones and at the same time, keep you healthier than if you just were spending your time chugging milk every day.

Healing Inflammation: There are several ways that inflammation affects the life of seniors and nothing is more pronounced than the inflammation that occurs due to arthritis. The pain from these joint issues is something that restricts mobility and as your mobility is restricted, your quality of life will diminish very quickly. Getting rid of inflammation from a proper diet is much better for you than taking anti-inflammatories that can cause lots of problems with your kidneys and your liver.

The Keto Diet does a great job of naturally reducing the anti-inflammatories; thanks to reducing the number of cytokines that are put in the body. When there are fewer cytokines, what will happen is that inflammation will lessen, and the joints will be looser and more mobile.

Deficiencies with Specific Nutrients: There are several different nutrients that people who are older have trouble with. The good news about ketosis is that it positively affects the different processes in your body. One of the first things that you need to rectify is iron deficiency. The problem with a lack of iron is that your brain will not be functioning all that well. You could get what is called brain fog and it is much easier to suffer from fatigue when you lack iron. Ketosis is something that will make sure that you get the right amount of iron so that your brain is operating at peak efficiency.

To that end, Vitamin B12 is something that is really important as well. Having high levels of Vitamin B12 helps prevent different debilitating neurological conditions like dementia. When you have high levels of Vitamin B12, this means that you will have a better chance of preventing the problems that come from Alzheimer's or Lewy Body Dementia, all thanks to the Keto Diet. Fats are important to have as well – they make sure that you have great skin and vision along with keeping your vitamin levels high. Also, having the right amount of fats is important for making sure that you are having exceptional cognition as you get older. Vitamin D deficiency also causes problems with cognition as well, and it also increases the risk of heart disease and cancer. It has been proven that the Keto Diet and the process of ketosis increases the levels of Vitamin D in your system, which in turn means that the risk of these problems goes down. The idea that you could lower your risk of heart disease, cancer, and remain sharp is tied to your diet should be motivation enough to do the Keto Diet.

Finally, one thing that is easy to see and is a common threat is that animal protein that is found in the Keto Diet is a great source for all of these nutrients. The bottom line is that people can get exactly what they need from the Keto Diet, especially seniors. Closing these nutritional gaps is imperative to have a great quality of life.

Regulating your Blood Sugar Levels is a theme that has been hammered home many times already in this book, but the bottom line is that your blood sugar is really critical to your quality of life. When you have unregulated blood sugar, this is something that can cause problems with the risk of Alzheimer's and Parkinson's Disease. There are several risk factors that come with this.

For example, if you are excessively eating carbs that include fructose, you are basically daring your brain to develop neurological conditions. It has been proven that the Keto Diet and ketosis lowers your blood sugar, and that in turn lowers the risk that you have from getting these particular different neurological disorders. The insulin response of the body is something that has been talked about a lot, and when your blood sugar is out of control with diabetes, that means your insulin is not doing the job it needs to do. So, if you are on the Keto Diet, this means your insulin is working the way it should and that your memory is something that will also be protected. Look, the worst stereotype about getting old is that your mind starts slipping. So, if you are in a position where you could change your diet and remain as sharp as ever, there is really no reason to avoid the Keto Diet. If anything, seniors should embrace it for this reason alone.

How the Keto Diet and Ketosis Is Important for Aging

The thing about the foods on the Keto Diet is that they deliver a ton of great nutrition and are packed with nutrients. If you have heard of superfoods, well, the Keto Diet is all about leveraging the food you eat for maximum benefit. The basal metabolic rate – also known as the minimum number of calories that are needed each day for survival – is less for seniors. But even though seniors need less calories than their younger counterparts, they do need the same amount of nutrients, and that is a place where the Keto Diet is of great assistance.

The reality is that people who are age 65 and older will not have an easy time living on junk food the way they could when they were younger. The body does not snap back the way it once did, and that is why seniors need to be more conscious about the food they are putting in their bodies. The food needs to support their health and fight disease. This is where the quality of life is found, and where they can enjoy the years that they worked to get to. Why not spend them in enjoyment instead of being in pain and torment because your diet is compromising your ability to enjoy yourself. The reality is that seniors cannot have empty calories in their bodies from sugar and food that have anti-nutrients laden throughout them.

The reality is that fats and proteins that are rich in nutrients are what will make sure that people who are seniors can live their best life because the calories that they are taking in are being used by the body in the most efficient way, and are not filler calories that would come from junk food. Furthermore, the food that is chosen by people who are older and are in different settings like a hospital or other clinical areas usually fairly brutal in terms of delivering the right amounts of nutrients. There is very little to gain from white bread, prunes, pasta, puddings, mashed potatoes, and other things that have lots of filler but little in the way of food that is actually good for you. The reality is that the government agencies that talk about the nutrition that you need are all about promoting a diet that is high in carbohydrates. The problem there is that this diet is not the one that is good for your long-term health. The reality for many people is that when they follow the standards that are published, they end up feeling less healthy and that in turn makes them feel worse for the wear.

This means that there is a greater level of cognitive decline and worse health. So, when going with the Keto Diet, what ends up happening is that ketosis helps people who are older get the nutrition that they need in order to make the most of their senior years instead of suffering through them and lamenting how they can't do what they did when they were younger. This is not how anyone intended to live in their retirement.

Using Ketosis to Achieve Longevity

The reality is that diet is a great way to improve your quality of life and when you are thinking about the rest of your life, do you want to live in comfort or do you want to enjoy what you are doing today for pain and discomfort in the future. The reality is we all should spend our time taking care of ourselves when we are younger so that we can enjoy the time when we are older. The bad news is that not everyone will use this high level of foresight. What they will do though, is do the right thing with their bodies as they get older, and the Keto Diet is a great way to repair some of the damage that has been done over the years. The good news here is that making the changes that support a healthy weight, lower blood sugar levels, proper immune system health, and a high level of cognition will help get all the way to the optimal level of health. Therefore, when you are a senior and you have a chance to really make the most of your golden years, and all it takes is having a diet that is all about your needs, is there any reason why you would not take advantage of this diet.

CHAPTER 5: KETOGENIC DIET AND WORKING OUT

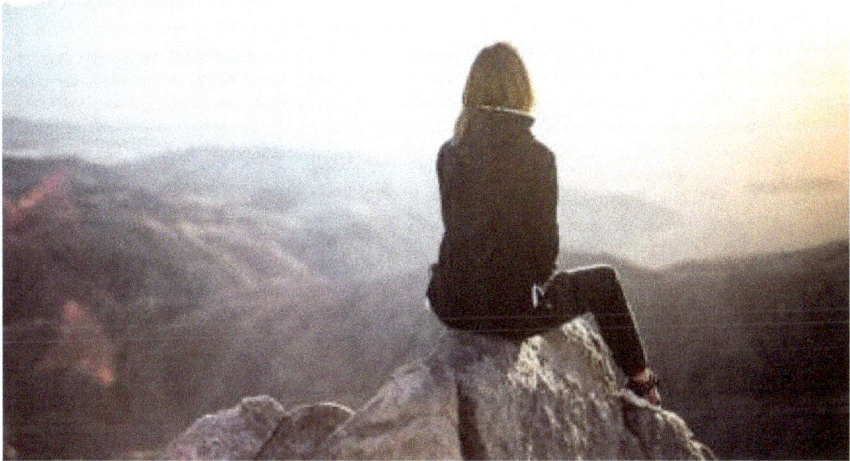

So, it's your first day at the gym; your goal is simply to get in shape and start living a better life. You walk into the gym; what is the first thing you do? Go lift in the squat rack? Maybe do some dumbbell/kettlebell work? Most likely, the first thing and the only thing that you would be doing is the treadmill or any piece of cardiovascular training. Don't get me wrong, cardiovascular training is not bad by any means, but in my opinion, your primary focus in the gym should be on the resistance training; you don't really need a gym membership to jog/walk as you can go for a jog/walk even without the use of treadmill by simply stepping outside. I understand that people who live in colder areas might not have the same privilege as someone living in a tropical area to go for a run outside year-round, but the point that I am trying to bring across is that your main focus walking into a gym should be on resistance training, rather than cardiovascular training; but that doesn't mean you should neglect cardiovascular training either. Cardiovascular training needs to be done at least two to four times a week, depending on people's goals and needs.

I know for some people, walking into the gym for the first time can be intimidating; you don't want to appear like you have no idea what you are doing here and be judged by fellow members, and you certainly don't want to do exercises with weights because you are not sure about them. In order for you to get to your goals, you will have to go thru that learning curve which needs to be started the day you walk into the gym. Looking up instructions online on how to do these exercise is not that hard; it barely takes any time to get the cue's and movement pattern down. The main key is to practice them, making sure you are using lighter weights and performing the exercise slower, so you feel the muscles that you are trying to work are indeed working.

If you do resistance training in this fashion for two to four weeks; three times a week of working out will teach your muscles to "fire" properly, and you will prime yourself to be doing exercises in a proper manner. Another way you can make sure you are doing your exercises right is by recording yourself performing it, then critiquing yourself based on the video you took performing that exercise. This method will give you a clear-cut idea of where your form is breaking down, and then you can go ahead and fix the issues that you are facing with that movement. If your form and technique are great, your risk of injury will go down significantly, and this is where you want to be at when you eventually get into more heavier weights; heavier meaning anything you will be performing for eight to ten reps and actually failing at the eight to ten rep range. I can't stress how important your first two weeks in the gym is; before you start getting yourself into a program, make sure you take two weeks or however long it takes to learn and perform exercises properly; but the main exercises you need to focus on are Pushing movement (push-ups), Pulling movement (Rowing movement), Hinging movement (deadlift), Squatting and Planks (core).

I will be talking about these five movements and how to perform them. These five movements are crucial, and should be in everybody's training plan. Whether you are a twenty-year-old trying to get big, or a fifty-year-old woman who is working out simply for health reasons, the first thing you should learn is these five movements, as these are the most difficult to learn and perform properly. However, after you have managed to learn them, you will be in a lot better position to start incorporating other exercises. Now since you have gotten an idea as to how you should be starting with regards to resistance training, let's move on to Cardiovascular training.

The best way to start doing cardiovascular training, in my opinion, is just walking. Walking is one of the best methods for you to get started with; it's easy, and its really low intensity can also be really relaxing for some. Cardiovascular training should be done by everyone, whether your goal is muscle gain or to lose body fat; doing cardiovascular training won't make you lose muscle. If done right, it will actually help you recover from workouts, which will help you recover from the higher volume of training which will also help you put on more muscle in a shorter period of time. There are a lot of other ways of doing cardiovascular training, but we won't get into that in this book, as there will be another book simply on cardiovascular training and how to get the most out of it based on fat loss and other stuff.

Resistance Training is Key

I talked about how resistance training can be beneficial for anyone. Whether you want to put on muscle, lose fat, or just stay in shape, it is crucial that you have resistance training in your program. Now let us get into the specifics of what resistance training is, and why you should be using it. Resistance training in layman's term, is a form or a type of exercise that you use for muscular strength and endurance. Now, let us get into the whys, and if your goal is to put on muscle, you need to achieve micro-tears in order for your muscles to grow stronger and bigger, this process is called hypertrophy. If your goal is to get in shape or lose weight, having a greater amount of muscle fibers will raise your metabolism, which will help you burn more energy at rest, meaning fat and glycogen. If you're a fifty-year-old woman who just want to stay in shape, resistance training will help you gain strength.

Now hypothetically speaking, if you tripped over and fall with no one around to help you get back up on your feet, you need strength to push yourself up off the floor. When you're young, that's the last thing you are worried about, but as you get older something as easy as this could be a struggle. If you can't get yourself up off the floor, and no one is there to help you, guess what? You're in trouble, and the sooner you start working on your strength, the better. That doesn't mean you need to train like a bodybuilder. You just need to do some type of resistance training to stay at an optimal health level.

Now let's talk about resistance training for people looking to put on muscle; for someone who is trying to put on as much muscle as possible, more volume is the key. Usually, after a workout, people's recovery is about forty-eight to seventy-two hours. That is depending on stress, sleep, nutrition, and genetics; but an average is forty-eight to seventy-two hours to recover from a workout. So, if you have gone online and looked up workout programs for bodybuilding, most of them are one to two body parts split, and you only train the muscle group once a week; that's a hundred and sixty-eight hours you have not trained that specific muscle. So, the conclusion is that you can train a certain muscle multiple times a week, which means you will put on more muscle and get stronger and faster than someone who only trains that specific muscle once a week. Programming is going to be more than one body part a day, unlike a bodybuilding split, and will be repeated a couple of times a week for someone who has the time for it. Three to five times a week would be perfect for them to achieve their goals in terms of putting on muscle; if not, then full-body workouts three times a week with higher intensity (heavier weights) can be used to yield similar effects. The main focus here is to train those muscles every two to four days making sure we are fully recovered first.

Now, for someone who is in their mid-fifties trying to get in shape because your doctor told you to or you have decided to embark on this journey yourself, then the resistance training part will be a lot more different for you than someone who is just trying to get bigger and muscular. Our main focus for someone who wants to stay healthy and get in shape is to gain strength, and start firing muscles that we have not used before and started putting on some muscle so we can actually achieve the first two things listed here. For people with the needs listed above, the best way to get to your goals will be full-body training, meaning all your major muscles in one day. Don't worry, as it doesn't take longer than one hour to do so. You should perform these workouts three times in a week; main goal for this is to make sure we are using slow tempo, meaning that we are performing the exercise in a slow fashion and making sure we are actually firing the right muscle fiber. At first it would seem like it's hard to actually fire the exact muscles you are trying to fire. However, if you consciously think about that muscle to "fire," eventually you will start to feel it; that is, if your form is correct. Take your time with your technique first. Don't overlook it. That goes for anyone.

Sets, Repetition, Tempo

Let me explain to you what exactly, sets, repetition and tempo is. Sets- how many times you perform an exercise before moving on to the next exercise. Repetition- How many times continuously you perform the exercises without any break. Tempo- How fast or slow you perform a rep. These three components are the single most important aspects of your training. You need to make sure you are actually following the rest set and tempo according to your training age, and your goals. If someone is in peak health and is an experienced trainee, then I would not make him wait five minutes before we get into our next set.

Unless we are training heavy or going to attempt a one-rep max, and if that's the case, then rest till we are fully recovered from going into the exercise.

Another thing that factors in when it comes to the three components is what your goals are, and what type of training you are into or doing right now. If your goal is to get lean and build up your cardiovascular health, then shorter breaks with a fast tempo and a couple of sets will work better for you to yield those results. Whereas we look at a different spectrum, if your goal is to put on the most muscle as possible, then time under tension is the key. This means that we will have to slow down the tempo and make the rest in between longer, and do multiple sets of the exercise to yield those results. There is no cookie-cutter rest, sets, and tempo that will do for any type of workout. People who have been training for a while tend to need a lot less rest in between than someone who is just starting to work out, since it's a new stimulus for them.

Reading Tempo Breakdown

Now let me show you the breakdown and how tempo is to be read in a workout template. If someone writes for example 2:0:2:0 in a workout template, and for example you are doing a push up; this would mean that two seconds down would be the lowering portion of the eccentric. The second number would mean a pause at the bottom or in the middle; the third would be the pushing up or the concentric portion of the repetition, and the final would be at the top of the repetition. If there is a hole at the top or in the middle, it should be specified where the hold is, in the middle or top/bottom. So this is how you would read how tempo is to be read. If the program has "x" in the tempo, it means lift as explosively in that lifting phase as you can.

Tempo Breakdown for Beginners

For someone who is just beginning to workout, go slower on the eccentric (on the way down) and a little bit faster on the concentric (on the way up). The reason why is so that we can start firing the right muscle fibers because in the beginning stage of working out, people tend to compensate other muscles fiber that they use most often. So, doing it slow something like 4:0:1:0 tempo would be a lot more beneficial for you.

How Sets Are Used for Different Goals

Sets are not so tricky as reps and tempo. Nonetheless, it is still important that they are used correctly towards your goal. Now basic sets scheme is three sets, which can be used in a beginner/ intermediate lifter/ trainee who wants to put on some muscle. But if you're an advanced lifter, three sets might be the thing of the past. Let's talk about how sets should be used for a beginner who is stepping in the gym for the first time. 1-2 sets per exercise with a sufficient amount of break.

Do that for 2-4 weeks, depending on how you feel, and then you can slowly start doing two exercises in the same sets back to back. This will build more muscle endurance and give your muscles more time under tension. I would not recommend doing this if you are about to perform a really big compound movement like bench press, squat, or deadlift, as the exercise itself is taxing enough. If you back to back, it will only make your sets moving on weaker, especially if you're training for strength. Then just focus on your major movements first, and then for your accessory movement, back to back exercises can be done. If your goal is hypertrophy and you have been working towards the goal of putting on some muscle for about a year or so, then back to back sets can really be beneficial for someone who is training towards that. It provides time under tension and you are able to add more exercises in your workout, which equals more volume. That's major when it comes to hypertrophy for bodybuilding. For someone trying to get strong, higher sets and lower reps would be the way to go; so higher intensity meaning heavier weights and lower reps.

Primal Movements

Most people workout because they want to put on muscle, or they want to lose some fat, and some just want to work out to get in shape and live a healthier life. All the scenarios above need to be doing something called a primal movement. These movements all together workout your whole body in such a manner that these movements will not only help you get stronger or give you that aesthetic look that you're going for, but this will also help your day to day life; hence it is known as a primal movement. Normally there are four primal movements, but personally, with years of experience in this field, I have decided to make it five primal movements, so here they are 1.Squat 2.Inverted rows/Trx rows (either works and can be adjusted to your physical capacity) 3 Push-ups/ modified push-ups 4. Hinge/ modified deadlift 5. Planks/ Abdominal work (depending on your fitness level).

All these primal movements can be modified to be accessible for anyone with any fitness level. Let us just say you cannot do push-ups off the floor. What you can do to make this movement more accessible to you is by doing it off your knees; meaning instead of your toes you can use your knees as a pivot point or use a bench or a squat rack with a barbell and have your torso more upright or in an elevation. This will make it easier for you to perform a push up. That goes with any primal movement. All of them can be modified to fit your needs. If primal movements are getting easy for you, then we can also make it harder by adding some resistance and/ or elevating it. Making an exercise easier is what we call a regression, and making an exercise harder is what we call progression. It doesn't matter if you are really advanced or just simply a beginner. Primal movements are to be performed to reach optimal results, whether it is for living a healthier life, or you simply want to add that extra pound of muscle. These movements are really powerful tools, and should be used correctly for individual needs, and be done safely. Now I will go thru all the primal movements with you and teach you the regression and progressions to this exercise, as I go through that with you.

Squat Regression to Progression

Let's start with regression if you cannot perform a bodyweight squat; what you start with is something called a box squat. Simply squat back like you are sitting back onto a chair, and then with one second, pause onto the box and get back up into a standing position. A proper squat would be when your knees and your hips are below 90 degrees when you look at it from the side. If that's hard for you to achieve even with a box, then start with a higher box or chair. Sit back on it and get back up and repeat that for sets and reps until its starts to feel like a 5 out of 10 in terms of how difficult it is. Then to progress from that, do the same thing but lower the box or get a smaller chair. Keep doing that until you have managed to get below 90 degrees. Now when going past 90 degrees on your box squats and it starts to feel easy, then instead of pausing, just tap the box and get back up rather than fully sitting on to the bench. This will feel a lot harder; eventually when it starts to feel like a 5 out of 10, then you should be able to do bodyweight squats. If you can't, then regress back to box squats with the tap and keep doing that until it feels like a 3 out of 10, and then try out bodyweight squats.

Now, when bodyweight squats start to feel like a 5 out of 10, then we can slowly start using some resistance to make it more challenging for you, so one of the ways you can make this challenging is by performing something called a goblet squat. Basically, it is about holding a kettlebell or dumbbell, and you hold it up to your chest level with both of your hands. If this description doesn't explain the exercise properly, there are a lot of videos online that will show you how to perform them in a detailed manner. If you don't have access to any kettlebell or dumbbell, then you can wear a backpack, and you load the backpack up with some heavier things lying around at your disposal; something like a heavy textbook or bottle of water. When you are capable of doing more than 45 lbs of kettlebell, dumbbell, or any weight form used on the squat for reps, then we can perhaps get into a safety bar squat or a barbell back squat; which one you move to depends on your shoulder mobility.

Rowing/Pull-ups Regression to Progression

Rowing is pretty easy to regress and progress from; the first thing you can start with is band rows or machine rows. Whatever you have available to you, start light and slowly up the resistance, whether it be bands or machine rows. When you have managed to row about 3/4 of your bodyweight for 10 reps using machine rows or bands, then you should be able to do an inverted rows. If you are using bands as resistance but you don't know what's the resistance in pounds, then get up to the heaviest band you have and row that for 10; and then try inverted rows (you should be able to get it done); beware as there are bands with insane resistance, so don't take banded rows lightly. When you are able to do inverted rows, you should be closer to doing a pull up; if you can complete a full bodyweight pull up, great. If not, here are a couple of things you can do. If you have a pull up assisted machine, you can use that. Start with a weight that you can do pull-ups with for 10 to 12 reps, and when it starts to feel like a 5 out of 10, then lower the weight, so you get less resistance. Then repeat the same process until you can do a pull up.

Let's say you don't have access to Pull up assistance machine; what you can do is use bands to make it easier for you. Simply hang the band in the middle of the pull up bar, or if you have a pull up bar with different grips, then just hang it on to the handle that you aren't going to be using. Now from there, simply get one of your knees onto the band and start doing pull-ups. This will help you get some resistance from the band, which will make it easier for you to do a pull up. The same principle applies as assisted pull up machine; go to a lighter band when it starts to feel like a 5 out of 10; at the end you should be able to do a pull up. Now, let's just say you don't have access to bands or pull up assistance machine. In that case, you can do something known as eccentrics. All you need to is simply get at the top of the pull up bar by using a chair or something elevated to get you to the top without any effort. From there, slowly lower yourself and repeat the process. Combine this with other back excises to strengthen your back, and then you should be able to complete a pull up.

Push-Ups Regression to Progression

Same as rows; push-ups should be easy to regress and progress from if you can't do a push up off the floor. Here are a couple of things you can do to make it happen. If you have access to a squat rack and a barbell, what you can do is simply do push-ups from an elevation; meaning place the barbell on the latches that the squat rack has on them and then simply do push-ups from there so your torso is elevated. This will make it easy for you to do push-ups. Let's say you can do push-ups off number 13 on the squat rack riser; keep doing that until it feels like a 5 out of 10 in terms of how hard. It then lowers the latch; keep doing that until you can do a push up off the floor. Now let's just say you don't have access to a squat rack, simply do push-ups off your knees and use that as your pivot point instead of your toes. When it feels like a 5 out of 10, then you should be able to do a push-up.

If you can't even do push-ups off your knees, what you can do is do more exercises that strengthen shoulders, triceps, and chest, and then try doing push-ups off your knees you should be able to eventually.

Hinge/Deadlift

The main thing in the deadlift/ hinge is not to squat the movement. Instead, hinge it. I see a lot of people do this movement incorrectly for a lot of reasons; their lower back is rounding, or they are squatting the weight instead of performing a deadlift. There are a lot of other faulty movement patterns that can be causing poor form in the deadlift/hinge, but we will cover the basics. What does it mean to hinge instead of squatting? Simply put, push your hips back. Believe it or not, a lot of people tend to have issues pushing their hips back and leaning your torso forward while keeping your back straight could be a lot of reasons; but one of them could be gluteus and hamstring tightness, which you should be working on in order to achieve a great deadlift/hinge.

Now since we have gotten that first exercise covered, it will progress us to a proper deadlift, which is kettlebell/ dumbbell. We will be using a riser or a stool to which you will be touching your kettlebell/ dumbbell to as you are leaning your torso forward and pushing your hips back; meaning that the stool will be behind you and low enough for you to bend your torso forward while keeping your back flat. Depending on your fitness and mobility level, adjust the height of the riser/stool.

So best cue for a deadlift/hinge would be:

1. Stand up straight with a kettlebell or dumbbell feet shoulder-width apart or slightly wider; whatever you feel comfortable doing.

2. Bend your knees softly and have the pressure on the middle of your foot.

3. Push your hips back while keeping your arms as close to your body as possible and keep the elbows straight, not bent.

4. Touch the riser, which is behind you. Start off like that and slowly lower the riser height to the point where you are touching the kettlebell/ dumbbell off the floor. Keep your back flat making sure you are pushing your hips back instead of squatting, and if you have issues keeping your back flat and you can't seem to bring the level down of your riser while keeping your back flat, it could be your gluteus and hamstrings are tight. Therefore, look up some stretches on YouTube or Google it, and most of you should be able to progress to a lower riser or stool after that. After following the steps listed above, you should be ready to move into a Barbell/Trap bar deadlift.

Planks/Abdominal Work

Day 1

1. Push-Ups (based on your fitness level)

2-3 sets of 12 to 15 reps

Tempo- 4:0:2:0

Rest- 30 to 60 seconds

2. Hinge/deadlift (based on your fitness level)

2-3 sets of 12 to 15 reps

Tempo- 4:0:2:0

Rest- 30 to 60 seconds

3. Trx/inverted row (Based on your fitness level)

2-3 sets of 12 to 15 reps

Tempo- 4:0:2:0

Rest- 30 to 60 seconds

4. **Squats** (Based on your fitness level)

2-3 sets of 12 to 15 reps

Tempo- 4:0:2:0

Rest- 30 to 60 seconds

When you are performing the squats, push-ups, and rows, you are using a lot of your core as theses exercise require you to be stable throughout the movement. Therefore, in my opinion, a lot of core/Abdominal training is required; if you are performing abdominal exercises for aesthetic reasons, planks might not be your go-to. Now let us keep it simple; if you have a big gut, I would not recommend doing planks as it can put a lot of pressure on your lower back if you try and hold it for a longer period of time. When you perform push-ups, you are working out your core; for someone with big gut, push-ups is fine for plank substitute. I would recommend doing something like crunches or leg raises instead. Do your primal movements, and when you have managed to reduce your gut, you can go ahead and perform some planks.

If you are on the chubbier side, you can do planks, but if you are on the side of being obese and your gut comes out a lot, that's when you shouldn't be performing planks; just wanted to clear that out. Now, let's talk about progression and regression. If you are starting off and you do have a bigger gut, start off with leg raises/ crunches; either works. I would recommend more doing of leg raises as it is easier on your spine, but either works just to make sure your spine is flat as you can keep it on your way up. Start with 5 - 10 reps, and when it starts to feel like a 5 - 10, add extra 5 more reps so on and so forth. Now for planks , start off with however long you can; hold the plank for let's say 30 seconds, and when the 30 seconds starts feeling like a 5-10, go up to 45 seconds and keep doing this until you can hold a plank for 2 minutes After that is achieved, add more weight to your back to make it harder.

Resistance Training for General Population

I have noticed that most of the books these days that are based on fitness, tend to be more advanced. By that, what I mean is books will talk about how to deadlift and squat properly when they don't realize most of the readers need to learn the basics first. It's like trying to build a house with no foundation; guess what, it will break with no foundation. Same thing with someone who starts of doing exercises like squats or deadlift with no foundation to support it. That's when perfecting primal movements come in to play in order to build foundation, so you can eventually get into a proper deadlift without hurting yourself. Therefore, you see the importance of training the right muscle fibers to get them to fire a certain way, so that when you move into the primal movements you are ready to roll. That being said, previously, I went into full detail on primal movements and how to progress to a squat, deadlift and all the other primal movements. I will make an example of three day a week workout plan for you guys, which you can follow to build a foundation and move into more of the advanced movements and workout plans, and actually reap the benefits out of it instead of hurting yourself.

As always, with your knowledge after reading this book, you can make your own workout routine and build that foundation. This Example workout is best suited for absolute beginners, although a lot of people who have been working out for some time can use it to get better results in a more advanced workout routine. This plan might look basic to some, but trust me to do this or similar template; using the knowledge you have acquired from this, you will most likely not injure yourself when you move on to a more advanced workout routine and actually see more results from the more advanced plan you follow in future. The best way to follow this plan is one day on one day off rule; so if you do day one on Monday, then do day two on Wednesday and then day three on Friday. Therefore, I highly recommend taking one day off between workouts, especially for "newbies." Although this book has been written by a certified trainer, please perform all these exercises at your own risk as there is no professional eye to look at your form and technique. Another thing is that there are couple of exercises that are in this example workout plan that I didn't go thru in-depth; please do a quick search online and you will find the right way to execute them.

Day 1.

1. Seated Band/ Machine row (Based on your fitness level)

2-3 sets of 10 - 12 reps

Tempo- 3:0:3:0

Rest- 45 to 70 seconds

2. Squats (Based on your fitness level)

2-3 sets of 10 - 12 reps

Tempo- 3:0:3:0

Rest- 45 to 70 seconds

3. Incline dumbbell press (use weights based on your fitness level)

2-3 sets of 10 - 12 reps

Tempo- 3:0:3:0

Rest- 45 to 70 seconds

4. Gluteus Bridges (Start with bodyweight and start adding resistance as you go along

2-3 sets of 10 - 12 reps

Tempo- 3:0:3:0

Rest- 45 to 70 seconds

5. Planks (Based on your fitness level)

Two sets of 10 - 60 seconds again based on your fitness level

Tempo- Just hold

Rest- 45 to 70 seconds

Day 2.

1. Squats (Based on your fitness level)

1-2 sets of 20 - 25 reps

Tempo- 2:0:1:0

Rest - As short as possible

2. Pull up/Trx or inverted row

3-4 sets of 10 to 12 reps

Tempo- 2:0:1:0

Rest - 60 to 90 seconds

3. Hinge/deadlift (based on your fitness level)

2-3 sets of 10 -12 reps

Tempo- 2:0:1:0

Rest - 60 to 90 seconds

4. Push-Ups (Based on your fitness level)

1-2 sets of 20 - 25 reps

Tempo- 2:0:1:0

Rest - As short as possible

5. Planks (Based on your fitness level

Two sets of 10 to 60 seconds again based on your fitness level

Tempo- Just hold

Rest - As short as possible

This workout format, with different variations of primal movements that I have pointed out, will yield you results for a lifetime — giving you better health and longevity when it comes to lifting weights and working out.

CHAPTER 6: HOW TO MAKE THIS A LIFESTYLE

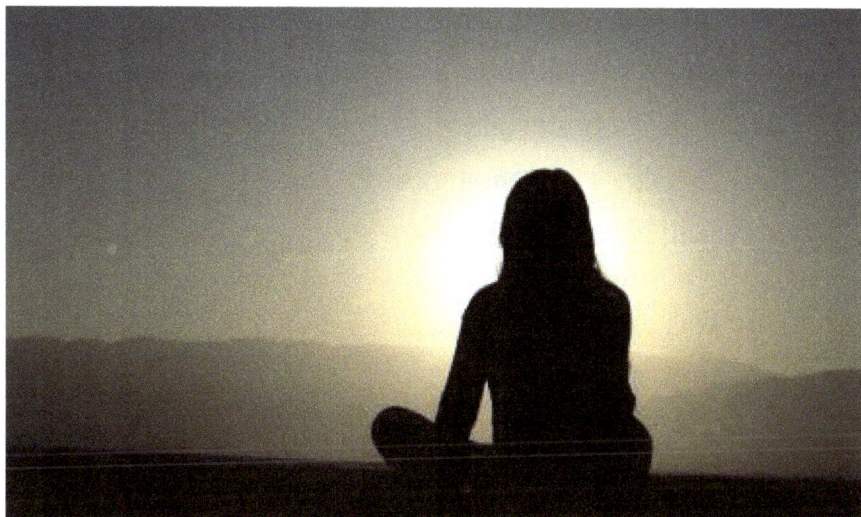

We will talk about what you should be doing, to make sure that you are not failing in your endeavors to start this diet to live a healthier life overall. This chapter will show you what you could be doing to make this diet your lifestyle, and to not only help you to start the Ketogenic diet and stay on track, but also to live with this eating plan for the rest of your life. These daily patterns will help you to not fail on your diet, and we understand that you might fail a couple of times in any diet, and it is understandable to do so. Nonetheless, this chapter will show you how to make sure you are consistent and not failing. These habits have been followed by many successful people to get optimal results in all of their aspects of life, whether it be fitness related or anything else. Make sure you start implementing all of these habits after you are done reading this book, as it will help you to make this diet your lifestyle. The reason why this chapter might sound philosophical is that the only way you will see success with this diet is if you do it consistently. For you to do that, you need to change your current lifestyle by being more productive and disciplined. You have to remember that healthy eating is more than just a meal; it's a lifestyle.

Plan Your Day Ahead

Planning your day ahead of time is crucial; not only does planning out your day help you to be more prepared for your day moving forward, but it will also help you to become more aware of the things you shouldn't be doing, hence wasting your time. Moreover, planning your day will truly help you with making the most out of your time. That being said, we will talk about two things 1. Benefits of planning out your day 2. How to go about planning out your day. So, without further ado, let us dive into the benefits of planning out your day.

It Will Help You Prioritize

Yes, planning out your day will help you prioritize a lot of things in your day to day life. You can allow time limits to the things you want to work on, from the most to the least. For example, if you're going to write your book and you are super serious about it. Then you need a specific time limit every day in which you work on a task wholeheartedly without any worries of other things until the time is up. Then you move on to the next job in line; so when you schedule out your whole day, and you give yourself time limits, then you can prioritize your entire day. The same thing goes for your diet; make sure you allocate time for prepping your meals for the next day, which will allow you to have meals ready for you when you need it, hence making it easy for you to continue on with your diet.

More Focus on the Task in Hand

This point is quite similar to the previous point, once you have started to plan out your day and you have become more aware of the things that you are about to do. With the time limit on all tasks that you do daily, it will create an urgency to get as much of the job done as you can before time is up, and you are moving on to your next appointment. This will help you to be more focused on the task at hand and get more things done. Many people consider healthy eating to be time-consuming, which it isn't if you prioritize your time the right way. If you cook your meals the day before and you set times for your meal, then it should not be a problem.

Work-Life Balance

You see, once you start planning out your whole day, you become more aware of your time and how to balance it out. Once you begin to write out your entire day ahead, you will know precisely what you are doing that day, so you don't have to do anything sporadically throughout the day. Always plan some time for yourself every day where you can wind down read a good book, meditate or maybe hang out with your friends and wind down. You will feel refreshed the next day; having to wind down and "chill out" will only make you a more productive person.

Planning out your whole day ahead will not only help you prioritize better. It will also help you be more focused on your task in hand and will help you have a better work-life balance. This also means that you are eating foods that you like once in a while; this will help you to stay motivated with the diet that you are following. So now that we have covered the benefits of planning out your day, let's dive into the how to's when it comes to planning out your day.

Summarize Your Normal Day

Now, before we start getting into planning out your whole day ahead, you need to realize that to plan your entire day, you need to know precisely what you are doing that day. Which means you need to write down every single thing you do on a typical day and write down the time you start and end; it needs to be detailed in terms of how long it takes for your transportation to get to work, etc.

Now after you have figured out your whole day, you can decide how to prioritize your day; moving on could be cutting out a task that you don't require or shortening your time for a job that doesn't need that much time. After you have your priorities for the day, you can add pleasurable tasks into your day like hanging out with your friends, etc.

Arrange Your Day

It is crucial that you arrange your day correctly, so the best way to organize your day is to make sure you get all your essential stuff done earlier in the day when your mind is fresh. After that's done, you can have some time for yourself to relax and do whatever it is that you want. Nevertheless, make sure you get all the things that need to be done before you can move on to free time for yourself. Another thing that will help you is to set time limits on each task, and once you start setting time limits, you will be more likely to get the job done.

Remove All the Fluff

What I mean by that is remove all the things that are holding you back from achieving your goals. Make sure you remove all of the things that are holding you back from getting the things that you need to be doing. If you have time for the fluff, do it; if not, then work on your priorities first. In conclusion, planning out your day will help you tremendously! Make sure you plan out your day every day to ensure successful and accomplished days.

Be Grateful

We will be talking about how to be grateful and what are the benefits of being thankful for what you have! Now believe it or not, being grateful every day will help you get more things done while keeping your mood elevated. See that you're thankful for the things you have, and you will start to feel like your mind will be in peace and joy. When your mind is in order and comfort, you will be more productive with all the tasks ahead of you that day. Being in a grateful state of mind will help you become less stressed and more positive, which will help your work quality by ten folds. So, it is pretty essential that you stay grateful not only for better work performance, but to also be in a peaceful state of mind. This will also help you to do more positive things with your diet, such as eat clean through the day. Let's discuss the three main benefits of being thankful.

1. Helps you start your day

Of course, if you start your day in a happy mood, you will more likely be keen to do more stuff and be more productive. If you read up on the most dedicated peoples and their day to day life, you will know that successful people tend to practice the same habits which I am going to be talking about in this chapter. The benefit of saying things you are grateful for, first thing in the morning will boost your positive vibes. When you talk about the things you're thankful for, you will complain a lot less and will not attract negative vibes, which is something we don't want! You always want to be in a positive mood as much as you can. To make sure you are in a positive vibe, write or say things you are grateful for.

2. You will become more approachable

Yes, being grateful will make you more approachable! Believe it or not, people do sense your "vibes" when you walk into the door. When you're more thankful for life, you are happier and more positive, which is what people want to be around with. Who knows; the next person you see could be an opportunity for you to grow your business or get a new job! So, always make sure you are in a great mood and counting your blessings still, as good things will come to you.

3. Lowered stress levels

I think this point is very self-explanatory. Let me ask you what most people are stressed about? Lack of resources; plain and straightforward. A lack of resources creates 99% of the stress. Once you start counting what you have rather than what you don't have, you begin to become a lot less stressed, which is suitable for your physical and mental health! So, make sure you always stay in a grateful mood. If you want to understand more about how being grateful can change your life, I recommend reading "The Magic" by Rhonda Byrne.

So, all in all, being grateful will help you live a better life and be more successful. Now you might be wondering how to be thankful throughout the day since it is so hard to block out ungrateful thoughts. Well, I'll show you three techniques that will help you combat your ungrateful thoughts and keep you in a grateful "vibe" most of your life.

Write ten things you are grateful for every morning:

You see, writing what you are thankful for will make your life a lot easier and help you start your day in gratitude. What I want you to do is first get a notebook/diary; then as soon as you wake up, I want you to write ten things you're grateful for. This could be anything from small as having water to drink to having a nice car; the whole point of this is to make you start your day in gratitude, as the way you start your day is the way your entire day is going to be most of the time. So, make sure to start your day on the right foot by writing down ten things you're grateful towards.

Don't forget the 1:5 ratio:

This is something I came up with, and it works great for me. You see whenever I say something I am angry or not grateful for, I always say five things I am super thankful for right after to get myself into the grateful "vibe" in the beginning; this method will be your best friend as it will save you from killing your "vibe."

Cut out negative people:

This task might be the hardest to do, but it is quite essential. See the people who you are around with are the people who will create your personality. Therefore, if you are around negative people, you will develop adverse circumstances for yourself; so if you are around people who are not upbeat about life and find everything wrong and never see the good in anyone, you need to cut them out and be around people who are happy and ready for what life has to offer. Now I get it, some cynical people can be your family members, and you can't cut them out; the best thing to do is 1. Make them understand what they are doing wrong 2. Show them how they can change their life, and if they still want to remain the same, then keep your distance.

In conclusion, it is essential that you are in a grateful "vibe" as it will not only help you with your mental and physical health, but it will also help you attract better people and better circumstances. Don't forget to practice the three methods we discussed in this chapter for you to be in a grateful 'vibe" throughout the day and life! That being said I hope this chapter shed some light on the importance of being grateful and how it can make or break your life, and I hope you don't take this chapter lightly. Being grateful is the most critical thing you can do to turn your life around. So be thankful!

Now that we have covered the part of being grateful, and how it can help you with your day to day life and eating habits, let us give you some concrete ideas on how to change the way you live your experience and to make it better.

Stop Multitasking

I think we are all guilty of this at a time, and if you are multitasking right now, I need you to stop. Now multitasking could be a lot of things, it could be as small as cooking and texting at the same time, or it could be as big as working on two projects at the same time. Studies are showing how multitasking can reduce your quality of work, which is something you don't want to do if your goal is to get the best result out of the thing that you are doing. That being said, there are a lot more reasons as to why you shouldn't be multitasking; so without further ado, let's dive into the primary reasons why multitasking can be harmful.

You're not as productive.

Believe it or not, you tend to be a lot less productive when you are multitasking. When you go from one project to another or anything else for that matter, you don't put all your effort into your work. You are always worried about the project that you will be moving into next. So, moving back and forth from one project to another will definitely affect your productivity. If you want to get the most out of your work, you need to be focused on one thing at a time and make sure you get it done to the best of your abilities. Moreover, you are more likely to make mistakes, which will not help you work to the best of your ability.

You become slower at your work.

When you are multitasking, chances are you will end up being slower at completing your projects. You would be in a better position if you were to focus on one project at a time instead of going back and forth, which of course helps you complete them faster. So, the thing that enables you to be faster at your projects when you're not multitasking is the mindset, and we often don't realize how much mindset comes into play. When you are going back and forth from one project to another, you are in a different mental state going into another project, which takes time to build and break. So, by the time you have managed to get into the mindset of project A, you are already moving into project B. It is always best that you devote your time and energy to one project at a time if you want it to do it at a faster pace.

It affects your creativity.

This is a significant disadvantage of multitasking, and studies are showing that multitasking can negatively affect your creativity. When something requires too much focus from your end, it becomes harmful to your creativity, and you need a lot more attention when multitasking compared to working on one thing at a time. If you want to succeed and live a better life, then you need to be creative, so if multitasking affects your creativity, then you need to stop doing that.

By now, you can see how multitasking can hinder the ability to work at your best. These three things listed above are a no-no when it comes to living a better and more productive life; not only does multitasking help not being prolific, but it makes you slower and less creative. So, all the benefits you thought you were getting multitasking was not accurate after all. Nonetheless, by now, you might be wondering how to go about working most efficiently. Well, the best way to put it is to work on one project at a time. I want you to put all your time and energy in the project you are doing currently and not worry about other projects. Make sure you set yourself goals when you start the project, which will help you be more efficient and faster at your work. so an example would be "you will not move on to another project until project A has been completed" or you have managed to hit a certain threshold at that specific project. So, to sum it all up.

- Do one project at a time

- Don't move on until it is completed, or you have managed to hit a certain threshold

- Set yourself a goal (time, quality, etc.)

All in all, multitasking will do you no good. It will only make you slower at your work and make you less productive. Making sure you stop multitasking is essential, as it will only help you live a better life. One thing to remember from this chapter is to put all your energy at one thing at a time, and this will yield you a lot of better projects or anything that you are working towards to be great. If you want to be more successful and live a better life, you need to make sure your projects are quality as I can't stress this point enough. You are probably reading this book because you want to get better at living your life or achieve goals that you just haven't yet. One of the reasons why you are not living the life that you want or haven't reached your goal could be a lot of things but, one of the items could be the quality of your work which could be taking a hit because of you multitasking. So, review yourself, and find out why you haven't achieved your goal and why you are not living the life that you want.

Then if you happen to stumble upon multitasking being the limiting factor or the quality of your work, I want you to stop multitasking and start working on one project at a time while giving it your full attention. What you will notice is that your work will have a higher quality and will be completed in a quicker amount of time following the steps listed above, which will change your life and help you achieve your life goals in a better more efficient way.

After reading this chapter, many might be thinking that this is more of a self-help book than it is a diet book. The truth is that we want you to understand how to live a better life by changing the habits that you are currently following. Truth be told, following a diet and making it a lifestyle is a lot more work than you think it is. For you to make it easy, you need to understand that you need to change your habits in order to be successful at this diet, which means you need to change the way you move, the way you think and the way you perform. This chapter gives you a clear idea on how to start living a better life by changing up your habits; once you do change your practices, you will notice that following the Ketogenic diet as a whole will be very easy for you. The reason why it will be straightforward for you is that you will change the way you move and change the way you live your life in general. Changing the way you live your life will not only help you get better results, but it will also help you to follow this diet as a lifestyle. Many people confuse diet as not being a part of a lifestyle, and it is something that they're supporting to better their health. But the truth is that when they're following a diet, they don't realize that it needs to be a lifestyle for it to be of health benefit. If you want to be healthier, then you need to make sure that you're taking care of your health 24/7 365 days a year.

This means you need to make this a lifestyle, and for you to make this a lifestyle, we need to understand some self-help techniques to keep it sustained for a more extended period. This is why this chapter is more self-help oriented; we wanted to make sure that this book is different from any other books that you've read when it comes to following the Ketogenic diet. The way we're going to be delivering it is by showing you how to change your lifestyle for the better instead of the worst. We're not just going to give you foods to eat and how to follow the Ketogenic diet, but in fact, we're going to change the way you eat overall, and to make it a better experience for you once you start getting into this diet. With that being said, I hope this chapter was be helpful to you, and we will see you in the next chapter.

Chapter 7: 10-Day Eating Plan + Recipes

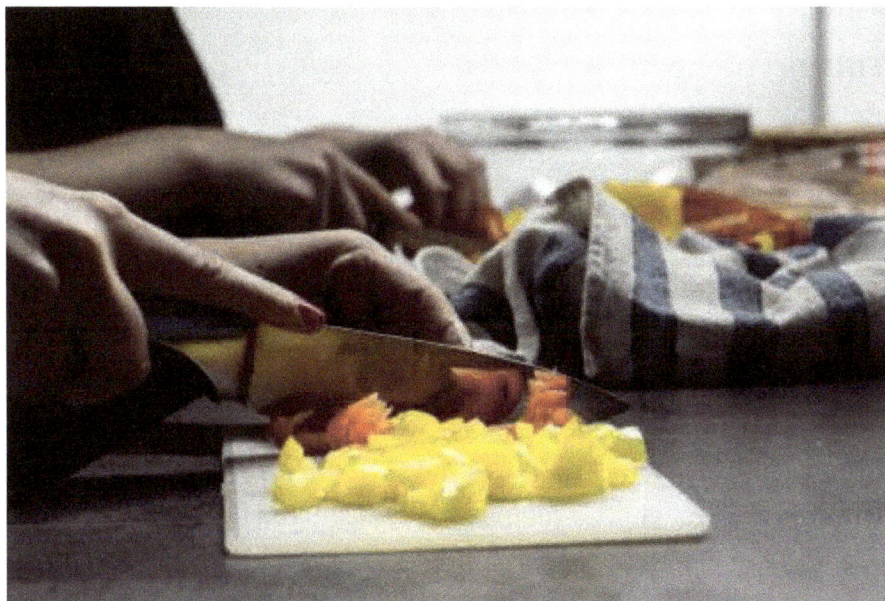

In this chapter, we will give you an excellent method to get you started. We will provide you with some of the most practical information you have ever used. Not only that, but we will also help you understand how to make a Ketogenic diet your lifestyle within ten days. Now, two things to remember when it comes to making the Ketogenic diet your lifestyle. Besides the fantastic recipes coming your way, you also need to have a great grocery list. We will give you the grocery list. Secondly, you need to have a basic understanding of macronutrients. One thing you need to remember would be that you will have to be in a caloric deficit regardless of what you think. If your goal is to lose weight, then you need to be in a caloric deficit. The only time you could get away with eating a little bit more would be when you follow intermittent fasting. That being said, here is a grocery list.

Things you need

1. Nuts (almond, cashews, peanuts)
2. Eggs
3. Meat (steak, pork)
4. Poultry (chicken)
5. Fatty fish (salmon etc.)
6. Low carb spices

You can always use the recipes for reference. However, these are just an essential grocery list for your Ketogenic diet. This will allow you to start having fun with the Ketogenic diet and seeing the results.

Now, the great thing about the Ketogenic diet would be that there is no requirement of you eating six meals a day. You can quickly get away with eating only three meals a day. Let us give you an eating plan to follow.

Breakfast: One of the breakfast recipes from the book

Lunch: One of the lunch recipes from the book

Snack: Handful of almonds

Dinner: One of the recipes dinner recipes from the book

This plan should be followed for ten days for you to see results. Two things to remember, the first thing would be that you need to count your macros, which is why we have provided you with macros on each meal. Secondly, make sure that you fight through the first ten days. This would be when the side effects subside. Now with that being made manifest, let us give you some fantastic recipes, which you can start following today to see better results in your health and wellness. Please make sure that you use these recipes in your diet, as they will help you to be more successful in your keto goals. The great thing about this plan would be the tasty meals you will get to have. You will forget that you are following the Ketogenic diet.

Breakfast

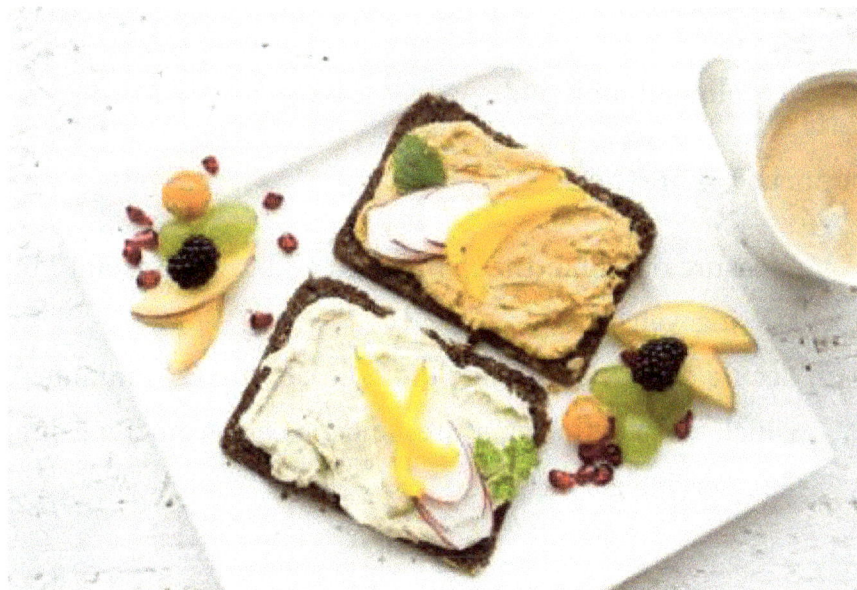

Almond–Chia & Coconut Pudding

Prep & Cook Time: 20 min.

Yields: 4 Servings

Nutrition Values: Calories: 130 | Fat: 12 g | Protein: 14 g |Net Carbs: 1.5 g

Ingredients:

- ¼ c. shredded coconut

- ½ c. of each:

o Chopped almonds

o Chia seeds

- 2 c. almond milk

Preparation Method:

1. Measure out all of the fixings and add to the Instant Pot, stirring well.
2. Secure the lid and select the high setting (2-5 minutes). Quick release the pressure, and place the pudding into four serving glasses.

Deviled Egg Salad

Prep & Cook Time: 30 min.

Yields: 5 Servings

Nutrition Values: Calories: 313 | Fat: 26.4 g | Protein: 16.4 g | Net Carbs: 1.3 g

Ingredients:

- 5 raw bacon strips

- 10 large eggs

- 2 tbsp. mayo

- 1 t. Dijon mustard

- 1 stalk green onion

- ¼ t. smoked paprika

- Pepper & Salt to taste

- Also Needed: 6-7-inch cake pan

Preparation Method:

1. Grease all sides of the pan that will sit inside of the pot on the trivet. Pour one cup of cold water in the bottom of the Instant Pot and add the steam rack.
2. Crack the eggs open in the pan (try not to break the yolks).
3. Place the pan on the rack. Secure the lid and set the timer for 6 minutes (high-pressure). Natural release the pressure and remove the pan.
4. Dab away any moisture. Flip the pan on a cutting board for the egg loaf to release. Chop and add to a mixing dish.
5. Clean the Instant Pot bowl and choose the sauté function (medium heat). Prepare the bacon until crispy.
6. Add to the chopped eggs with the mustard, mayo, paprika, pepper, and salt. Toss and garnish with green onion.
7. Serve the way you like it!

Egg Cups & Cheese

Prep & Cook Time: 15 min.

Yields: 4 Servings

Nutrition Values: Calories: 115 | Fat: 9 g | Protein: 9 g | Net Carbs: 2 g

Ingredients:

- 4 eggs

- ½ c. sharp shredded cheddar cheese

- 1 c. diced veggies—example, tomatoes, mushrooms, etc.

- ¼ c. Half & Half

- Pepper & Salt to taste

- 2 tbsp. cilantro—chopped

Ingredients for the Topping:

- ½ c. shredded cheese of your choice

Also Needed:

- 4 wide-mouthed jars
- 2 c. water

Preparation Method:

1. Whisk the veggies, eggs, Half & Half, salt, pepper, cheese, and cilantro.
2. Combine the mixture into each of the jars. Secure the lids (not too tight) to keep water from getting into the egg mix.
3. Arrange the trivet in the Instant Pot and add the water. Arrange the jars on the trivet and set the timer for 5 minutes (high pressure). When done, quick release the pressure, and top with the rest of the cheese (½ cup).
4. Broil if you like for 2-3 minutes until the cheese is browned to your liking.

Ketogenic Eggs

Prep & Cook Time: 20 min.

Yields: 4 Servings

Nutrition Values: Fat: 14.4 g | Protein: 7.3 g | Net Carbs: 8.3 g

Ingredients:

- 1 tbsp. chopped shallot

- 3 tbsp. ghee

- 1 sliced jalapeno—matchstick

- 1 t. of each:

  o Ground cinnamon
  o Cumin seeds

- 3 sliced garlic cloves

- 1 coarsely chopped green bell pepper

- 2 coarsely chopped tomatoes

- ½ t. of each:

  o Turmeric
  o Ground ginger

- o Salt

- ½ c. chopped cilantro

- 4 eggs—beaten

Preparation Method:

1. Add the ghee to the Instant Pot. Melt using the sauté function and add the cumin seeds, cooking until aromatic.
2. Continue cooking for 3 minutes along with the shallots. Stir in the peppers, tomatoes, jalapenos, and garlic. Sauté 3 additional minutes and add the salt, ginger, salt, and turmeric.
3. Whisk in the eggs and cook until set (30 seconds). When the eggs are at the right texture, sprinkle with the pepper, salt, and cilantro.
4. Secure the lid and prepare for 13 minutes. Quick release the steam and serve.

Lunch

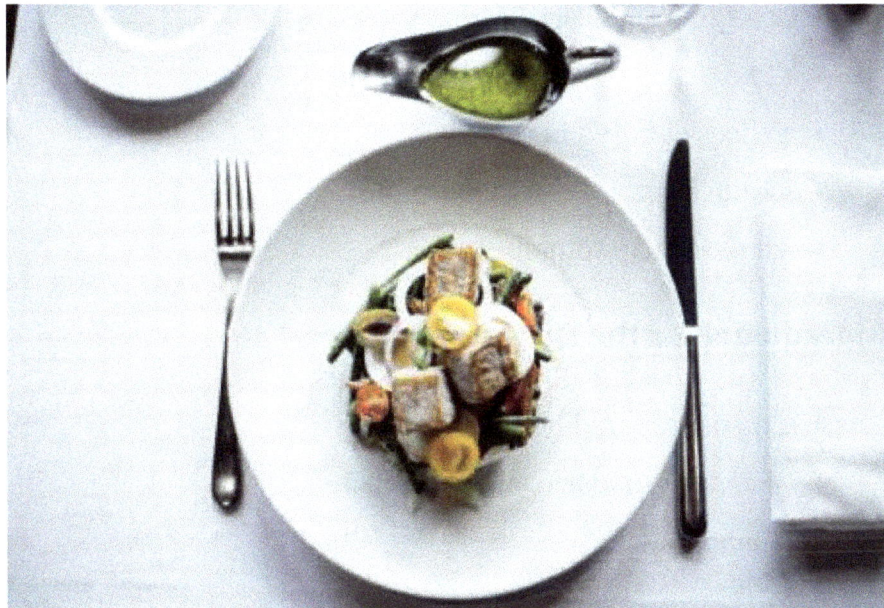

Salads

Bistro Steak Salad with Horseradish Dressing

Serves: 2

Nutritional Values Per Serving:

Calories: 736 | Protein: 41.4 g | Carbohydrates: 6.2 g| Fat: 59.4 g

Ingredients:

- 1 (12 oz.) rib-eye steak
- ¼ t. of each:
- Pepper

- Salt
- 1 (2.1 oz.) small red onion
- 1 (7 oz.) bag romaine salad greens
- 4 slices uncured bacon
- ½ cup (2 oz.) sliced radishes
- 4.2 oz. cherry tomatoes

Ingredients for the Dressing:

- 2 tbsp. prepared horseradish
- ¼ c. mayonnaise (see recipe below)
- Pepper and salt

Method:

1. Thinly slice the onion and radishes.
2. Place parchment paper on a baking tin. Set the oven temperature to 350°F. Arrange the bacon in a single layer in the pan. Bake for 15 minutes. Drain and break into small pieces.
3. Pat the steak with paper towels. Season with the pepper and salt. Grill for four minutes and flip. Continue cooking another 12-15 minutes (medium is approximately 12 minutes or internal temperature of 155°F.).
4. Let it cool down five minutes, and slice against the grain into small slices.
5. Prepare the dressing (below) and enjoy.

Low-Carb Mayonnaise for the Horseradish Dressing

Serves: 4

Nutritional Values Per Serving: Included with above recipe

Ingredients:

- 1 egg yolk
- 1-2 t. white vinegar/lemon juice
- 1 tbsp. Dijon mustard
- 1 c. light olive oil

Method:

1. Ahead of time, take out the egg and mustard to become room temperature.
2. Mix the mustard and egg. Slowly, pour the oil until the mixture thickens.
3. Pour in the lemon juice/vinegar. Stir well. Add a pinch of salt and pepper for additional flavoring.

Caprese Salad

Serves: 4

Nutritional Values Per Serving:

Calories: 190.75 |63.49 g Fat |Carbohydrates: 4.58 g | Protein: 7.71 g

Ingredients:

- 3 c. grape tomatoes
- 4 peeled garlic cloves
- 2 tbsp. avocado oil
- 10 pearl-sized mozzarella balls
- 4 c. baby spinach leaves
- ¼ c. fresh basil leaves
- 1 tbsp. of each:
- -Brine reserved from the cheese
- -Pesto

Method:

1. Use aluminum foil to cover a baking tray. Program the oven to 400°F. Arrange the cloves and tomatoes on the baking pan and drizzle with the oil.

2. Bake 20-30 minutes until the tops are slightly browned.

3. Drain the liquid (saving one tablespoon) from the mozzarella. Mix the pesto with the brine.

4. Arrange the spinach in a large serving bowl. Transfer the tomatoes to the dish along with the roasted garlic. Drizzle with the pesto sauce.

5. Garnish with the mozzarella balls, and freshly torn basil leaves.

Egg Salad Stuffed Avocado

Serves: 6

Nutritional Values Per Serving:

Calories: 280.57 | Fat: 24.83 g| Carbohydrates: 3.03 g| Protein: 8.32 g

Ingredients:

- 6 large hard-boiled eggs
- 3 celery ribs
- 1/3 med. red onion
- 4 tbsp. mayonnaise
- 2 tbsp. fresh lime juice
- 2 t. brown mustard
- Pepper & salt to taste
- ½ t. cumin
- 1 t. hot sauce
- 3 med. avocados

Method:

1. Begin by chopping the onions, celery, and eggs. Discard the pit and slice the avocado in half.
2. Combine with all of the other fixings except for the avocado.
3. Scoop the salad into the avocado and serve!

Thai Pork Salad

Serves: 2

Nutritional Values Per Serving:

Calories: 461 | Fat: 32.6 g| Carbohydrates: 5.2 g| Protein: 29.2 g

Ingredients for the Salad:

- 2 c. romaine lettuce
- 10 oz. pulled pork
- ¼ medium chopped red bell pepper
- ¼ c. chopped cilantro

Ingredients for the Sauce:

- 2 tbsp. of each:
- -Tomato paste
- -Chopped cilantro
- Juice & zest of 1 lime
- 2 tbsp. (+) 2 t. soy sauce
- 1 t. of each:
- -Red curry paste
- -Five Spice
- -Fish sauce

- ¼ t. red pepper flakes
- 1 tbsp. (+) 1 t. rice wine vinegar
- ½ t. mango extract
- 10 drops liquid stevia

Method:

1. Zest half of the lime and chop the cilantro.
2. Mix all of the sauce fixings.
3. Blend the barbecue sauce components and set aside.
4. Pull the pork apart and make the salad. Pour a glaze over the pork with a bit of the sauce.

Vegetarian Club Salad

Serves: 3

Nutritional Values Per Serving:

Calories: 329.67| Fat: 26.32 g| Carbohydrates: 4.83 g| Protein: 16.82 g

Ingredients:

- 2 tbsp. of each:
- -Mayonnaise
- -Sour cream
- ½ t. of each:
- -Onion powder
- -Garlic powder
- 1 tbsp. milk
- 1 t. dried parsley
- 3 large hard-boiled eggs
- 4 oz. cheddar cheese
- ½ c. cherry tomatoes
- 1 c diced cucumber
- 3 c. torn romaine lettuce
- 1 tbsp. Dijon mustard

Method:

1. Slice the hard-boiled eggs and cube the cheese. Cut the tomatoes into halves and dice the cucumber.
2. Prepare the dressing (dried herbs, mayo, and sour cream) mixing well.
3. Add one tablespoon of milk to the mixture - and another if it's too thick.
4. Layer the salad with the vegetables, cheese, and egg slices. Scoop a spoonful of mustard in the center along with a drizzle of dressing.
5. Toss and enjoy!

Pasta

Cauliflower 'Mac N Cheese'

Serves: 4

Nutritional Values Per Serving:

Calories: 294 | Fat: 23 g| Carbohydrates: 7 g| Protein: 11 g

Ingredients:

- 3 tbsp. butter
- 1 head cauliflower
- 1 c. cheddar cheese
- Black pepper & sea salt to taste
- ¼ c. of each:
- Unsweetened almond milk
- Heavy cream

Method:

1. Cut the cauliflower into small florets and shred the cheese.
2. Prepare the oven to 450°F. Cover a baking sheet with aluminum foil or parchment paper.

3. Melt 2 tbsp. of butter. Toss the florets and butter. Give it a shake of pepper and salt. Place the cauliflower on the baking pan and roast 10-15 minutes.

4. Warm up the rest of the butter, milk, heavy cream, and cheese in the microwave or double boiler. Pour on the cheese and serve.

Fettuccine Chicken Alfredo

Serves: 2

Nutritional Values Per Serving:

Calories: 585 | Fat: 51 g| Carbohydrates: 1 g| Protein: 25 g

Ingredients:

- 2 tbsp. Macadamia nut oil
- 2 minced garlic cloves
- ½ t. dried basil
- ½ c. heavy cream
- 4 tbsp. grated parmesan

Ingredients for the Chicken and Noodles:

- 2 chicken thighs - no bones or skin
- 1 tbsp. olive oil
- 1 bag Miracle Noodle - Fettuccini
- Salt and pepper

Method:

1. *For the Sauce*: Add the cloves to a pan with the butter for two minutes. Empty the cream into the skillet and let it simmer two additional minutes. Toss in one tablespoon of the parmesan at a time. Add the pepper, salt, and dried

basil. Simmer three to five minutes on the low heat setting.

2. ***For the Chicken:*** Pound the chicken with a meat tenderizer hammer until it is approximately ½-inch thick. Warm up the oil in a skillet using the medium heat setting and put the chicken in to cook for about seven minutes per side. Shred and set aside.

3. ***For the Noodles:*** Prepare the package of noodles. Rinse, and boil them for two minutes in a pot of water.

4. Fold in the noodles along with the sauce and shredded chicken. Cook slowly for two minutes and enjoy.

Lemon Garlic Shrimp Pasta

Serves: 4

Nutritional Values Per Serving:

Calories: 360| Fat: 21 g| Carbohydrates: 3.5 g| Protein: 36 g

Ingredients:

- 2 bags angel hair pasta
- 4 garlic cloves
- 2 tbsp. each:
- Olive oil
- Macadamia oil
- ½ lemon
- 1 lb. large raw shrimp
- ½ t. paprika
- Fresh basil
- Pepper and salt

Method:

1. Drain the water from the package of noodles and rinse them in cold water. Add them to a pot of boiling water for two minutes. Transfer them to a hot skillet over medium heat to remove the excess liquid (dry roast). Set them to the side.

2. Use the same pan to warm the oil, and smashed garlic. Saute a few minutes but don't brown.

3. Slice the lemon into rounds and add them to the garlic along with the shrimp. Saute for approximately three minutes per side.

4. Add the noodles and spices and stir to blend the flavors.

Pizza

BBQ Meat-Lover's Pizza

Serves: 2

Nutritional Values Per Serving:

Calories: 205| Fat: 27 g| Carbohydrates: 3.5 g| Protein: 18 g

Ingredients:

- 2 c. (8 oz.) mozzarella
- 1 tbsp. psyllium husk powder
- ¾ c. almond flour
- 3 tbsp. (1 ½ oz.) cream cheese
- 1 large egg
- ½ t. of each:
- Black pepper
- Salt
- 1 tbsp. Italian seasoning

Ingredients for the Topping:

- 1 c. (4 oz.) mozzarella cheese
- To Taste: BBQ sauce
- Sliced Kabana/hard salami
- Bacon slices

- Sprinkled oregano - optional

Method:

1. Set the temperature of the oven to 400°F.
2. Melt the cheese in the microwave until it melts – about 45 seconds. Toss in the cream cheese and egg, mixing well.
3. Blend in the psyllium husk, flour, salt, pepper, and Italian seasoning. Make the dough as circular as possible. Bake for ten minutes. Flip it onto a piece of parchment paper.
4. Cover the crust with the toppings and some more cheese. Bake until the cheese is golden, slice, and serve.

Beef Pizza

Serves: 4

Nutritional Values Per Serving:

Calories: 610| Fat: 45 g |Carbohydrates: 2 g | Protein: 44 g

Ingredients:

- 2 large eggs
- 1 pkg. (20 oz.) ground beef
- 28 pepperoni slices
- ½ c. of each:
- Shredded cheddar cheese
- Pizza sauce
- 4 oz. mozzarella cheese
- Also Needed: 1 Cast iron skillet

Method:

1. Combine the eggs, beef, and seasonings. Place in the skillet to form the crust. Bake until the meat is done or for about 15 minutes.
2. Take it out and add the sauce, cheese, and toppings. Place the pizza in the oven a few minutes until the cheese has melted. Remove and enjoy!

Bell Pepper Basil Pizza

Servings: 4 - 2 Pizzas

Nutritional values per serving:

Calories: 411.5| Fat: 31.32 g| Carbohydrates: 6.46 g| Protein: 22.26 g

Ingredients for the Pizza Base:

- 6 oz. mozzarella cheese
- 2 tbsp. of each:
- -Fresh parmesan cheese
- -Cream cheese
- Psyllium Husk
- 1 t. Italian seasoning
- 1 large egg
- ½ t. of each:
- Black pepper
- Salt

Ingredients for the Toppings:

- 4 oz. shredded cheddar cheese
- ¼ c. marinara sauce
- 1 med. vine ripened tomato
- 2-3 med. bell peppers
- 2-3 tbsp. fresh basil – chopped

•

Method:

1. Set the temperature in the oven to 400°F.
2. Melt the cheese in the microwave
3. \ until melted and pliable or for 40-50 seconds. Add the remainder of the pizza base fixings to the cheese – mixing well with your hands.
4. Flatten the dough to form the two circular pizzas. Bake for ten minutes. Remove and add the toppings. Leave for about 8-10 additional minutes.
5. Let it cool and serve.

Pita Pizza

Serves: 2

Nutritional Values Per Serving:

Calories: 250| Fat: 19 g| Carbohydrates: 4 g| Protein: 13 g

Ingredients:

- ½ c. marinara sauce
- 1 low-carb pita
- 2 oz. cheddar cheese
- 14 slices pepperoni
- 1 oz. roasted red peppers

Method:

1. Set the oven to 450°F.
2. Slice the pita in half and put on a foil-lined baking tray. Rub with a bit of oil and toast for one to two minutes.
3. Pour the sauce over the bread, sprinkle with the cheese, and other toppings. Bake for another five minutes or until the cheese melts.

Tacos & Wraps

Chipotle Fish Tacos

Serves: 4

Nutritional values per serving:

Calories: 300 | Fat: 20 g| Carbohydrates: 7 g| Protein: 24 g

Ingredients:

- ½ small diced yellow onion
- 2 pressed cloves of garlic
- 1 chopped fresh jalapeno
- 2 tbsp. olive oil
- 4 oz. chipotle peppers in adobo sauce
- 2 tbsp. each:
- -Mayonnaise
- -macadamia nut oil
- 4 low-carb tortillas
- 1 lb. haddock fillet's

Method:

1. In a skillet, fry the onion on med-high for five minutes.
2. Lower the temperature to the medium heat setting. Toss in the garlic, and jalapeno. Stir for another two minutes.

3. Chop and add the chipotles, along with the adobo sauce into the pan.

4. Drop the butter, mayonnaise, and fish into the pan and cook about eight minutes.

5. Make the Tacos: Fry the tortilla for approximately two minutes for each side. Chill and shape them with the prepared fixings.

Cumin Spiced Beef Wraps

Serves: 2

Nutritional Values Per Serving:

Calories: 375| Fat: 26 g| Carbohydrates: 4 g| Protein: 30 g

Ingredients:

- 1-2 tbsp. coconut oil
- ¼ onion – diced
- 2/3 lb. ground beef
- 2 tbsp. chopped cilantro
- 1 diced red bell pepper
- 1 t. minced ginger
- 2 t. cumin
- 4 minced garlic cloves
- Pepper and salt to your liking
- 8 large cabbage leaves

Method:

1. Warm up a frying pan and pour in the oil. Sauté the peppers, onions, and ground beef using medium heat. When done, add the pepper, salt, cumin, ginger, cilantro, and garlic.

2. Fill a large pot with water (3/4 full) and wait for it to boil. Cook each leaf for 20 seconds, plunge it in cold water and drain before placing it on your serving dish.
3. Scoop the mixture onto each leaf, fold, and enjoy.

Dinner

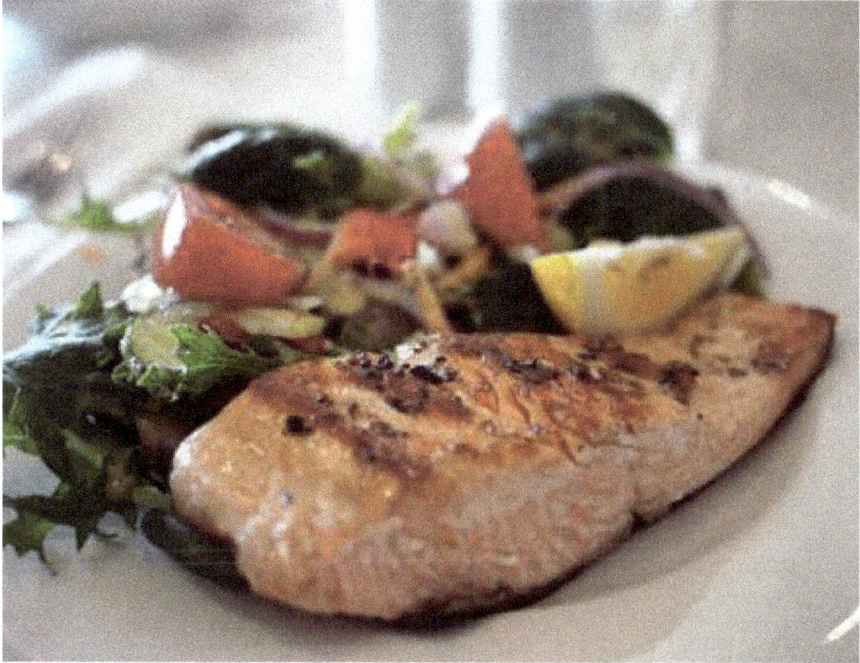

Beef for Dinner

Balsamic Beef Pot Roast

Serves: 10

Nutritional Values Per Serving:

Calories: 393 | Fat: 28g| Carbohydrates: 3 g| Protein: 30 g

Ingredients:

- 1 boneless (approx. 3 lb.) chuck roast
- 1 t. of each:

- -Garlic powder
- -Black ground pepper
- 1 tbsp. kosher salt
- ¼ c. balsamic vinegar
- ½ c. chopped onion
- 2 c. water
- ¼ t. xanthan gum

For the Garnish:

- Freshly chopped parsley

Method:

1. Combine the salt, garlic powder, and pepper and rub the chuck roast with the combined fixings.
2. Use a heavy skillet to sear the roast. Add the vinegar and deglaze the pan as you continue cooking for one more minute.
3. Toss the onion into a pot with the (two cups) boiling water along with the roast. Cover with a top and simmer for three to four hours on a low setting.
4. Take the meat from the pot and add to a cutting surface. Shred into chunks and remove any fat or bones.
5. Add the xanthan gum to the broth and whisk. Place the roast meat back in the pan to warm up.
6. Serve with a favorite side dish.

Cheeseburger Calzone

Serves: 8

Nutritional Values Per Serving:

Calories: 580| Fat: 47 g| Carbohydrates: 3 g| Protein: 34 g

Ingredients:

- ½ yellow diced onion
- 1 ½ lb. ground beef – lean
- 4 thick-cut bacon strips
- 4 dill pickle spears
- 8 oz. cream cheese – divided
- 1 egg
- ½ c. mayonnaise
- 1 c. of each:
- -Shredded cheddar cheese
- -Almond flour
- -Shredded mozzarella cheese

Method:

1. Program the oven to 425°F. Prepare a cookie tin with parchment paper.
2. Chop the pickles into spears. Set aside for now.

3. Prepare the Crust: Combine ½ of the cream cheese and the mozzarella cheese. Microwave 35 seconds. When it melts, add the egg and almond flour to make the dough. Set aside.

4. Cook the beef on the stove using medium heat.

5. Cook the bacon (microwave for five minutes or stovetop). When cool, break into bits.

6. Dice the onion and add to the beef and cook until softened. Toss in the bacon, cheddar cheese, pickle bits, the rest of the cream cheese, and mayonnaise. Stir well.

7. Roll the dough onto the prepared baking tin. Scoop the mixture into the center. Fold the ends and side to make the calzone.

8. Bake until browned or about 15 minutes. Let it rest for 10 minutes before slicing.

Nacho Steak in the Skillet

Serves: 5

Nutritional Values Per Serving:

Calories: 385.4| Fat: 30.67 g| Carbohydrates: 5.9 g| Protein: 18.87 g

Ingredients:

- 1 tbsp. butter
- 8 oz. beef round tip steak
- 1/3 c. melted refined coconut oil
- ½ t. turmeric
- 1 t. chili powder
- 1 ½ pounds cauliflower
- 1 oz. each shredded:
- -Cheddar cheese
- -Monterey Jack cheese

Possible Garnishes:

- 1 oz. canned jalapeno slices
- 1/3 c. sour cream
- Avocado – Approx. 5 oz.

Method:

1. Set the oven temperature to 400°F.
2. Prepare the cauliflower into chip-like shapes.
3. Combine the turmeric, chili powder, and coconut oil in a mixing dish.
4. Toss in the cauliflower and add it to a tin. Set the baking timer for 20 to 25 minutes.
5. Over med-high heat in a cast iron skillet, add the butter. Cook until both sides are done, flipping just once. Let it rest for five to ten minutes. Thinly slice, and sprinkle with some pepper and salt to the steak.
6. When done, transfer the florets to the skillet and add the steak strips. Top it off with the cheese and bake for five to ten more minutes.
7. Serve with your favorite garnish, but count those carbs.

Portobello Bun Cheeseburgers

Serves: 6

Nutritional Values Per Serving:

Calories: 336| Fat: 22.8 g| Carbohydrates: 4 g| Protein: 29.1 g

Ingredients:

- 1 lb. ground beef - lean 80/20
- 1 t. of each:
- 1 tbsp. Worcestershire sauce
- -Pink Himalayan salt
- -Ground black pepper
- 1 tbsp. avocado oil
- 6 slices sharp cheddar cheese
- 6 Portobello mushroom caps

Method:

1. Remove the stem, rinse, and dab dry the mushrooms.
2. Combine the salt, pepper, beef, and Worcestershire sauce in a mixing container. Form into patties.
3. Warm up the oil (medium heat). Let the caps simmer about three to four minutes per side.

4. Transfer the mushrooms to a bowl - using the same pan - cook the patties four minutes, flip, and cook another five minutes until done.
5. Add the cheese to the burgers and cover for one minute to melt the cheese.
6. Add one of the mushroom caps to the burgers along with the desired garnishes and serve.

Steak-Lovers Slow-Cooked Chili in the Slow Cooker

Serves: 12

Nutritional Values Per Serving:

Calories: 321| Fat: 26 g| Carbohydrates: 3.3 g| Protein: 38.4 g

With Toppings:

Calories: 540.3| Fat: 41.32 g| Carbohydrates: 13.49 g| Protein: 32.47 g

Ingredients for the Chili:

- 1 c. beef or chicken stock
- ½ c. sliced leeks
- 2 ½ lbs. (1-inch cubes) steak
- 2 c. whole tomatoes (canned with juices)
- 1/8 t. black pepper
- ½ t. salt
- ½ t. cumin
- ¼ t. ground cayenne pepper
- 1 tbsp. chili powder

Optional Toppings:

- 1 t. fresh chopped cilantro
- 2 tbsp. sour cream

- ¼ c/ shredded cheddar cheese
- ½ avocado – sliced or cubed

Method:

1. Toss all of the fixings into the cooker - except the toppings.
2. Use the cooker's high setting for about six hours.
3. Serve, add the toppings, and enjoy.

Vegetarian Keto Burger on a Bun

Serves: 2

Nutritional Values Per Serving:

Calories: 637| Fat: 55.1 g| Carbohydrates: 8.7 g| Protein: 23.7 g

Mushroom Ingredients:

- 1-2 tbsp. freshly chopped basil – 1 t. dried
- 2 medium-large flat mushrooms – ex. Portobello
- 1 tbsp. of each:
- -Coconut oil/ghee
- -Freshly chopped oregano – ½ t. dried
- 1 crushed garlic clove
- ¼ t. salt
- Black pepper

Serving Ingredients:

- 2 large organic eggs
- 2 slices cheddar/gouda cheese
- 2 tbsp. mayonnaise
- 2 keto buns – see recipe below

Also Needed:

1 griddle pan/regular skillet

Method:

1. Prepare the mushrooms for marinating by seasoning with crushed garlic, pepper, salt, ghee (melted), and fresh herbs. Save a small amount for frying the eggs. Marinate for about one hour at room temperature.
2. Arrange the mushrooms in the pan with the top side facing upwards. Cook for about five minutes on the med-high setting. Flip and continue cooking for another five minutes.
3. Remove the pan from the burner and flip the mushrooms over and add the cheese. When it is time to serve, put them under the broiler for a minute or so to melt the cheese.
4. With the remainder of the ghee, fry the eggs leaving the yolk runny. Remove from the heat.
5. Slice the buns and add them to the grill, cooking until crisp for about two to three minutes.
6. To assemble, add one tablespoon of mayonnaise to each bun and top them off with the mushroom, egg, tomato, and lettuce.
7. Put the tops on the buns (see recipe below) and serve.

Keto Buns for the Burger

Serves: 12

Nutritional Values Per Serving:

Calories: 189| Fat: 12.6 g| Carbohydrates: 3.1 g| Protein: 11.6 g

Note: Erythritol has 0.4 g carbohydrates, and Xylitol has 10 g.

Dry Ingredients:

- ½ c. of each:
- -Ground sesame/poppy seeds
- -Flax meal
- -Unflavored whey protein/egg white protein powder
- 1 c. of each:
- -Almond flour
- -Coconut flour
- 1 tbsp. of each:
- -Dried oregano
- -Minced garlic
- -Cream of tartar
- -Xylitol or Erythritol
- 2 tsp. baking soda
- 1 tsp. salt

Wet Ingredients:

- 2 large eggs
- 6 large egg whites
- 1 tbsp. extra-virgin coconut oil
- 2 c. hot water

Method:

1. Prepare the oven temperature to 350°F.
2. Toss the sesame seeds in a processor and pulse until powdery. Blend in all of the dry components, omitting the coconut flour for now. Mix well.
3. Combine the hot water and eggs. Add to the dry fixings, mixing well. Gradually combine the coconut flour until you have a dense uniformity. Be sure not to make the mixture too dry.
4. Scoop the dough onto a baking pan - leaving them several inches apart and sprinkle with the poppy/sesame seeds. Bake for 20-30 minutes or until browned.

Chicken for Dinner

Barbecue Pulled Chicken in the Slow Cooker

Serves: 8

Nutritional Values Per Serving:

Calories: 219| Fat: 7.2 g| Carbohydrates: 4.3 g| Protein: 33.8 g

Ingredients:

- 3 lb. chicken thighs
- 1 t. of each:
- -Cumin
- -Smoked paprika
- -Onion powder
- ¼ t. pepper
- ¾ t. salt - divided
- 1 t. maple extract
- ¼ c. apple cider vinegar
- 1 c. sugar-free ketchup
- ½ c. water
- ½ t. clear liquid stevia
- 1 tbsp. unsweetened cocoa powder
- ¼ t. cumin

Method:

1. Remove all of the bones and chicken and arrange the chicken on a baking sheet. Combine the salt, pepper, cumin, onion powder, and paprika together. Rub it over the chicken.

2. Pour the ketchup, vinegar, and water into the slow cooker. Stir, and add the rest of the fixings. Lastly, add the chicken.

3. Close the lid and cook four hours on high or eight hours on low.

4. Enjoy over some rice (add the carbs).

Chicken Parmesan

Serves: 2

Nutritional Values Per Serving:

Calories: 600| Fat: 32 g| Carbohydrates: 3 g| Protein: 74 g

Ingredients:

- 1 lb. breasts of chicken
- 2 tbsp. parmesan cheese
- 1 oz. pork rinds
- 1 egg
- ½ c. of each:
- -Marinara sauce
- -Shredded mozzarella

Possible Garnish Ingredients:

- -Pepper and salt
- -Garlic powder
- -Oregano

Method:

1. Program the oven temperature to 350°F.

2. Use a food processor/Magic Bullet to crush the pork rinds and parmesan cheese. Add them to a bowl.

3. Pound the chicken breasts until they are ½-inch thick. Beat the egg and dip the chicken in for an egg wash. Dip the chicken into the crumbs.

4. Arrange the breasts on a lightly greased baking sheet. Sprinkle with the seasonings and bake 25 minutes.

5. Dump the marinara sauce over each portion. Garnish with the mozzarella and bake for 15 minutes.

6. Enjoy with a bed of spinach.

Coconut Curry Chicken Tenders

Serves: 5

Nutritional Values Per Serving:

Calories: 494 | Fat: 39.4 g| Carbohydrates: 2.1 g| Protein: 29.4 g

Ingredients for the Tenders:

- 1 large egg
- 1 pkg. chicken thighs (24 oz.) deboned with skin /5 thighs
- ½ c. of each:
- -Crumbled pork rinds (1 ½ oz.)
- -Unsweetened shredded coconut
- 1/2 t. coriander
- 2 t. curry powder
- ¼ t. of each:
- -Onion powder
- -Garlic powder
- Pepper & salt to your liking

Sweet and Spicy Mango Dipping Sauce Ingredients:

- ¼ c. of each:
- -Sour cream
- -Mayonnaise
- 1 ½ t. mango extract

- 2 tbsp. sugar-free ketchup
- ¼ t. cayenne pepper
- ½ t. of each:
- -Ground ginger
- -Garlic powder
- -Red pepper flakes
- 7 drops liquid stevia

Method:

1. Set the oven to 400°F.
2. Whisk the eggs and debone the thighs. Slice them into strips (skins on).
3. Add the spices, coconut, and pork rinds to a Ziploc-type bag. Add the chicken, shake, and place on a wire rack. Bake for about 15 minutes. Flip them over and continue baking for another 20 minutes.
4. Combine the sauce components and stir well. Serve with your piping hot chicken tenders

Pizza Chicken Casserole in the Slow Cooker

Serves: 3

Nutritional Values Per Serving:

Calories: 228 | Fat: 8.8 g| Carbohydrates: 6 g| Protein: 31.2 g

Ingredients:

- 2 cubed chicken breasts
- 1 can tomato sauce – 8 oz.
- 1 t. Italian seasoning
- 1 bay leaf
- Dash of pepper
- ¼ t. salt
- To Garnish: ½ c. shredded mozzarella cheese
- Recommended: 2-quart slow cooker

Method:

1. Remove the bones from the chicken and chop into cubes. Add them to the slow cooker.
2. Pour in the sauce over the chicken and add the spices. Stir and cook on the low setting for three to four hours.
3. Serve with the cheese as a garnish.

CONCLUSION

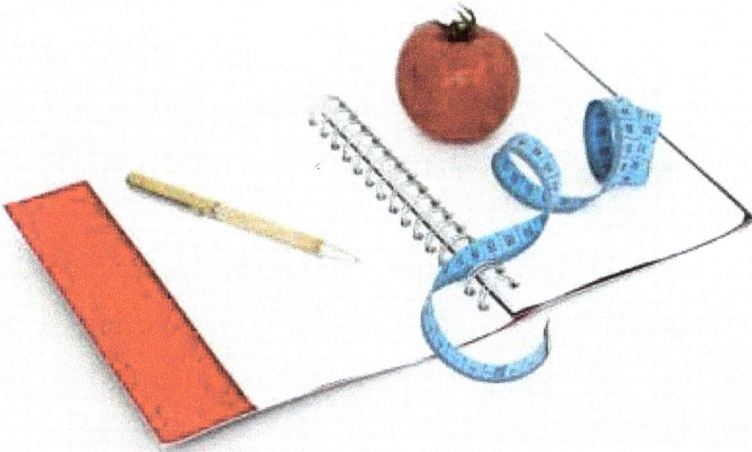

Thank you so much for making it all the way to the end of this book. We hope that you have found a treasure trove of information, which is certain to help you keep those unwanted pounds off. Best of all, you don't need any special science or equipment. You have everything you need in order to make the best of your personal abilities to follow this eating plan.

Indeed, the road to health and wellbeing has its ups and downs; in fact, we all go through them. There is no arguing about that. However, what truly counts is your motivation and desire to stay on track despite any drawbacks. We sincerely hope that attitude has been come across throughout this book.

Please go over this book again, as repetition is the best way in which we are able to learn. Before you know it, you will be an expert in the arts of the ketogenic diet. Best of all, you will be able to share your knowledge with your friends, family and colleagues. You will surely be able to help them improve their overall health and wellbeing, just like you have.

If you feel that this book has been useful and informative, do tell your friends and family about it... or anyone you think would be interested in this topic. The more we are able to tell people about the benefits of the ketogenic diet, the more we can help others improve their health and wellbeing.

What could be better than that?

Thanks again. Hope to see you in the next one.

www.ingramcontent.com/pod-product-compliance
Lightning Source LLC
Chambersburg PA
CBHW050727030426

42336CB00012B/1446